THE
MENOPAUSE MONOLOGUES
II

More real experiences by real women

Compiled by Harriet Powell

Cover and illustrations by M.R. Goodwin

First Printing 2020

The Little Taboo Press

ISBN 9781916139121

Foreword by Shelter

Shelter is honoured to be supported through this book and welcomes the opportunity for women's experiences of the menopause to be heard. We work to ensure that all voices are listened to in terms of homelessness and bad housing and could not be more pleased to be associated with this publication.

Shelter was founded in 1966 to act upon the inequalities and poor provision of housing. Sadly, our services are needed more than ever over fifty years on. We provide advice, support and guidance to people who are homeless, facing homelessness or experiencing bad housing, through our telephone and web chat, face-to-face support and range of legal services. We campaign for a future where everyone has a right to a safe home. We are a charity and rely upon support to keep our services and work going. We simply would not be able to do this without our fantastic supporters.

Thank you to Harriet, and to everyone who has made this book a reality.

Lindsay Tilston Jones

Introduction

Wow! What a journey it's been, from that first lightbulb moment ("Why not publish a collection of menopause stories?") to the completion of this second volume. I have been overwhelmed by the number of inspirational women who have wanted to contribute.

As with the first book, the sheer range of experiences is breathtaking: for some, the menopause is very clearly a nightmare – a litany of sleepless nights, low mood and lost libido (and that's just for starters) – while others seem to breeze through it. But regardless of where they lie on the spectrum, it is the honesty of these accounts that truly shines through. It's hard to open up and be vulnerable, but it is so refreshing and reaps such rewards: in sharing our vulnerabilities, we invite closeness and compassion.

When I was collecting stories for the first book, I assumed everyone would want to be anonymous. After all, the menopause involves some pretty personal stuff. And I was right: that's what all bar one of the contributors requested. This time round things were different. A whopping 80% of the stories you are about to read are published under their authors' real names. And though I think no less of the handful who have chosen to remain anonymous, I can't help feeling that's progress. It suggests to me that we're starting to get better at talking about the menopause, and that slowly but surely we are breaking the taboo. If these two little books help in any way to continue the trend, that will be job done. Read on – and enjoy the ride!

Jennifer's story

(Jennifer Kennedy, author of *Galloping Catastrophe: Musings of a Menopausal Woman*)

Many women express frustration that their significant others don't understand what they're going through when it comes to the menopause – and are therefore about as much use as a chocolate teapot at giving support.

If you want your partner to empathise with you fully, then the best plan is to get them to live twenty-four hours as a menopausal woman. This immersion should give them real insight into how you feel.

Simply ask them to follow these guidelines:

- Start the experiment at about 10pm. Go to bed with a thermal vest, four jumpers with hot water bottles between each layer, and keep your electric blanket on full.

- Once you are soaked through with sweat, get up and change the bedclothes and yourself. Try not to wake your partner while doing this. Repeat at least three times during the night.

- Ensure you have a recording of all the things you are worried about. Set your alarm for 3am and listen to it for two hours.

- Just before you are about to fall asleep again, stick a bag of midges or mosquitoes in bed with you and lie itching and scratching for an hour or so.

- Get up and wear clothes that are a size too small around the waist. Get really annoyed with your socks.

- Before going to work, tweeze your beard rather than shave.

- Smoke five joints and take two sleeping tablets – plus a swig of that cold remedy that makes you sleep lots. This might just get you some way to understanding the 'brain fog' symptom.

- At work, nip to the kitchen every couple of hours (and always before key meetings with your boss) and stand in front of the industrial-sized ovens for a full ten minutes.

- Halfway through meetings, think of something very, very sad and try to hold back the tears. If someone annoys you, tell them to shut up and then worry about it for the rest of the day.

- Go to the toilet every half-hour.

- If you laugh or sneeze, ensure you wee yourself a bit. Choose whether to wear a bulky incontinence pad or risk a wet patch on your trousers.

- About 3pm, go to the toilet again, lie on the floor and have a little snooze.

- After your nap, pick up a family-sized bar of chocolate and scoff the lot to give you the energy to get through the rest of the day.

- In the evening, allow your partner to rub your genitals with coarse sandpaper for a long, long time. Finally, fake an orgasm so that you can get on with watching the latest box set in bed with a bottle of wine.

- This should help you gain a full understanding of what the woman in your life is going through. If it isn't sufficient to get you to modify your behaviour around her, then repeat for approximately twelve years.

Elizabeth's story

Menopause hit my vanity first. It began with a photograph of me out with friends – only something wasn't quite right. Was that me, or Elizabeth I in one of her wigs? I couldn't tell.

The more I stared at the photo, the more I realised it was my hairline that was wrong. It was further back than it should have been. Strange. Must have been how I was holding my head. Except the next photo showed the same thing. And the next. And then, looking in the mirror, I could see a distinct patch. Oh my God, a bald patch!

I went to the doctor, who kindly informed me I had male pattern baldness – yes, honestly – and ordered blood tests for my iron levels before informing me that if there was nothing wrong with them (there wasn't), there was nothing they could do.

So I changed hairstyles.

A few months later, I began getting pains in my legs. Pains that felt as if my very marrow was being tortured. Pains so strong they woke me up.

I went back to the doctor (a different one in my surgery, this being the NHS) and he prescribed vitamin D.

"How are you otherwise?" he asked. "How's your general wellbeing? Periods still coming?"

"Oh, that side of things is absolutely fine," I replied. "Haven't had one for months now. I feel fantastic. It's just these aching legs."

"Are you still sexually active? You could be pregnant…"

Cue a sprint to the pharmacist for a pregnancy test. On New Year's Eve. Followed by relief.

But the vitamin D seemed to do its job and my aches dropped to bearable levels. I mean, didn't everyone my age say "Ooof!" when they stood up because of their sore joints? And slouching over a computer all day was bound to make my shoulders tense…

Fast-forward several months and I was training for the Great North Run. I'd got up to ten miles without stopping – a major miracle for a woman who was always last at cross-country at school – but every now and then, I'd get small heart palpitations. They never happened when I was running – far from it, I felt strong and powerful then – but when I stopped, I'd get a flutter just strong enough to make me put my hand to my heart to try and quell it.

The GP ordered me to stop training and have a stress test, a procedure in which you are wired up to a heart monitor whilst on a treadmill.

I'd committed to doing the GNR to raise money for Guide Dogs, and not being able to train (and not knowing if I'd even be able to compete) really wasn't helping the anxiety I was feeling at times.

The palpitations and the anxiety freaked me out so much that I ended up in A&E one night after work, convinced that I was having a heart attack. After several hours, the lovely doctor basically asked if it was a family trait to 'worry' about health and sent me on my way, adding that he saw no reason why I shouldn't get back to training.

As my husband and I walked home, I fretted non-stop about wasting the doctor's time and adding to the strain on the NHS. I also made a mental note to double-check everything I'd done at work that day. Double-checking my work was beginning to become the norm. Triple-checking, even. I'm a journalist: a job I love. But I was starting to worry that I was losing my touch. Young people would arrive at meetings with their laptops, whilst I'd come armed with my notebook and a cup of tea. What an antique they must think me...

And then there was the occasion I didn't spot a mistake until it went live on our website. What if it happened again, and this time we were sued? Fine, so the only person who had spotted it hadn't thought it was worth mentioning – but this riled me even more.

In fact, getting angry was becoming more and more normal. Bloody people on the Tube who wouldn't move to let you out; bloody politicians; bloody influencers; bloody so-called-friends on social media; bloody husband; bloody family; and BLOODY TUDOR CRISPS FOR NO LONGER MAKING GAMMON FLAVOUR.

I started to wake up at 2am, angry at somebody I felt had slighted me, or a news story, or myself. I went from 'live and let live' to wanting everyone to hurt. A lot.

When I wasn't angry, I was worried. Frantically worried that something bad was going to happen. Fear gripped me so tightly that I couldn't breathe at times. Then I'd berate myself. What a drama queen! How dare I feel down when I had a roof over my head and others were sleeping on the streets? No wonder people were talking about me behind my back! I had to pull myself together...and I would, once I had a bit more energy. I must be eating badly to be so constantly tired. Even my fingers were fatigued. And itchy. My whole body was itchy. Perhaps I was missing some vitamins...

But at least I no longer had to worry about periods. God, the menopause really was wonderful, wasn't it? Periods vanishing for months on end – it was a bit of a bummer when they returned, true, but they were very light and no longer painful, so I couldn't complain – and yeah, these hot flushes were a bit of a drag, but I didn't get too many and so long as a window was open, I was fine. Loving it… Yes, the hot flushes were growing in number and sometimes left me having to stop what I was doing, but that was alright. It was simply the menopause and I was, after all, a hypochondriac. The A&E doctor had said so, hadn't he? I bet he was telling everyone about the bloody stupid woman he'd had in one night…

Then I was hit by a two-day battering of debilitating hot flushes – and my husband took to the internet. And THAT was when I discovered what the menopause truly was, that night when he found a symptoms-checker and discovered that everything I had been going through for the last three or four years was on it.

The hot flushes, itchiness, rage, paranoia, fear, aches, palpitations, hair loss – it all had one simple answer. Menopause. And I had never known.

It was a lightbulb moment that, once I had started HRT, I wrote about for my blog, *50Sense.net*. The response was amazing – and still is. All these months on and I still get so many women (and their husbands, partners and families) writing to say they felt just the same way. And, like me, they'd never known it was all menopause-related.

That's why I joined forces with two other women to begin the Pausitivity KnowYourMenopause campaign. We want posters displaying menopause symptoms in every GP surgery and health centre in the UK.

Too many women have contacted me to say that they, too, were ignorant of what menopause could entail (apart from the hot flushes and irregular periods). And none of them was aware of the psychological symptoms.

Women need to know what menopause can mean, and so does the rest of society, because how we feel impacts on all those around us. By highlighting symptoms on a poster, we can break the taboo that stops us talking about the menopause and empower women to have the sorts of conversations they need to be having.

Looking back on my 'menopause self', I feel as if I'm viewing a different person. It's hard to believe that scared, frightened, tired, angry woman was me. I have my ups-and-downs – we're still trying to find the right HRT combination – but most days I feel good. Some days I feel bloody invincible. If this is what life is like postmenopause, then bring it on!

Most of all, though, I feel passionately that no one should have to go through what I did. I'm channelling all my menopause strength into making life better for the next woman. And so long as I'm doing that, I don't feel as if the last few years of suffering have been in vain.

Flo's story

So, when is this thing properly going to kick in? My mum had a hysterectomy, so I can't use her as a gauge. I haven't had children: does that affect it? I suppose it'll just happen when it's ready.

Throughout my forties, my periods were pretty regular and not particularly heavy. I experienced discomfort on the first day of my cycle, and a couple of days of irritability leading up to the bleeding, but I could live with it. This year is the first time I've noticed that changes are afoot. I'm 52, I've started to miss the odd period and it is affecting me both physically and mentally.

The first sign was a burning mouth. It felt like I had scalded it and it was painful to eat. I looked it up online and found that it was a symptom of the menopause. I also read that it was sometimes due to a deficiency in vitamin B12, so I bought some and the burning subsided after a couple of weeks. I still find it uncomfortable to eat or drink anything acidic, and spicy food (which I used to love) isn't pleasant anymore. I often have a metallic taste in my mouth and I'm constantly thirsty.

I am also permanently angry. I feel irritable and impatient with everyone and have to make a real effort to be nice. I won't put up with things I used to tolerate, and I speak my mind more than I used to. But then again, the world is a pretty frustrating place at the moment, so maybe it's not irrational to be angry…

I am tired. It comes in waves. Afternoons are particularly bad. I often just want to close my eyes. It takes longer to recover after sport, though having said that, sport is still something I do quite a bit of. I was concerned about developing osteoporosis, so I've introduced more jumping around and weight-lifting – but my main thing is cycling. It seems to clear my head. I have several sporty friends who have menopausal symptoms and it's been interesting to swap stories and to hear that we are all experiencing it differently.

I am itchy. I thought it was chlorine that was causing the problem, but I haven't been swimming for a while and it's still there. It's not a big deal, just something else that's new. If I miss a period, it tends to come right on time the following month, and then the symptoms subside. I may bleed again two weeks later, and then four weeks after that. The bleeding seems to help relieve my symptoms of PMS for a few weeks, especially the mood and energy-related ones.

I started to read all I could about the menopause – but stopped because so much of it felt negative or scary. So far, my symptoms have been very manageable, so I'm just ploughing on and taking it month by month. However, I do believe that reading about other people's experiences can validate what you are going through, and that's why I wanted to contribute to this book. I hope my story helps someone. Writing it has certainly helped me: I can see I've had quite an easy time of it!

Jane L's story

(Jane Lewis, author of *Me and My Menopausal Vagina*)

One of the many symptoms of the menopause is vaginal dryness. This makes it sound like a minor inconvenience: a bit like a sore throat, solved by a good old British cup of tea. If only…

The official term for it is Genitourinary Syndrome of Menopause, which certainly gives it more of the gravity it deserves, though I don't much like the word 'syndrome'. It implies it's all in our heads, when in truth it's down to declining levels of oestrogen. I think 'syndrome' should be replaced with 'symptoms', because that's what GSM is: a catalogue of symptoms which many women experience, of which vaginal dryness is just one.

My name is Jane Lewis and I am 53. I have suffered from every symptom of GSM since the age of 45 (whilst still having periods): vaginal dryness (causing chafing whilst walking); a burning vulva; thinning/atrophying skin of the vulvar area; painful or impossible sex; old episiotomies almost splitting open; itching; watery discharge; the inability to wear underwear or jeans; the inability to sit down for long; the inability to ride either a bike or a horse. See what I mean? 'Vaginal dryness' doesn't quite cut it.

Pretty much overnight, I went from being an active horse-rider to an almost-suicidal married mother-of-three. For a short time, I hid away due to the shame and taboo surrounding the condition, and also due to the constant burning. (The soreness of the vulva and bladder drives you mad and darkens the brightest of days.)

What's so shocking is that I am not a rarity. GSM affects about 60% of women, and that figure is considered conservative, since many of us are self-treating and (surprise, surprise!) putting-up and shutting-up.

I have become a campaigner for the change that must happen – and through raising awareness, I have opened a massive can of worms. Women mustn't suffer in silence. They must be given a voice. That grumpy old lady sitting on a rubber ring, wearing pads day and night and smelling of urine? One day that could be you. I have spoken to enough healthcare practitioners to realise that this is A Very Big Problem. We are postmenopausal for potentially thirty years, and GSM often rears its ugly head just when we thought we had 'sailed' through it all. (Oh, how I hate that saying!)

I want all women, including my three daughters and granddaughter, to be educated about GSM, and about the menopause in general. The medical profession needs to take these subjects far more seriously, because women's sex lives and relationships are being ruined. Wearing incontinence pads isn't normal during the menopause: you should be able to laugh without peeing your pants, you shouldn't be getting repeat UTIs and you shouldn't be getting up several times a night to use the toilet.

Together with my daughter, Penny, I have written a book about it: *Me and My Menopausal Vagina*. I am determined that other women don't have to suffer like I have.

Julie's story

I am 48 and now nine months into the year-long trek towards full menopause. It feels like it's come a bit early, but hey ho!

I've searched numerous websites for lists of associated symptoms and realise now that I've been perimenopausal since shortly after giving birth to my daughter. For four years after my pregnancy my periods were normal, but sometime around my daughter's fifth birthday I started experiencing short gaps between them (approximately 22 days) and very heavy loss. This meant I had to change feminine care every couple of hours. It zapped my energy levels, and some days were a real struggle: it felt like I was wading through treacle. Then, about two years ago, the length of time between periods increased to 33-35 days, with less heavy flow. I had mood swings and chronic PMT-like symptoms. After that I started skipping whole cycles. This was incredibly tricky as I never knew when I was due on.

When the hot flushes were at their peak, I would wake up in the night feeling clammy and uncomfortable. Luckily, that time has passed, but my sleep pattern has changed considerably. I now get about six hours of proper sleep. There's no point going to bed early, as it makes me feel more tired, not less!

My weight has stayed static, but the fat distribution has changed. My chest size has increased, and I have more tummy fat, but less fat on my hips. This means I need to look at what exercise I do to combat the shape-change and stay healthy. Cue a fitness app to track weight, calories and exercise. I don't have any scales at home, so am logging everything and watching to see if the way I feel in my clothes changes. I have always found that the biggest incentive to losing weight is to be able to buy smaller-sized clothes, rather than staring at the needle on the scales. I now eat foods with more calcium and iron in. I can't even begin to tell you how much raw spinach I consume!

My taste buds have also changed. I can't tolerate nearly so much sugar and prefer savoury foods. I'm no longer a chocoholic and can't stand meringues unless they're accompanied by berries. I don't like cola, and diet drinks have become a no-go area.

I have read countless articles about osteoporosis and osteoarthritis and am starting to think hard about what multivitamins I might need to take. I have considered HRT, but the risk of breast cancer and ovarian cancer has put me off for family history reasons.

My hair feels thinner. I will have to consider changing my style. I also need to think about facial creams to protect my skin, especially because I suffer from vitiligo. And I will definitely have to revamp my make-up bag. The products I have used for years are now no longer appropriate. I need concealer for the vitiligo and a different shade of foundation to enrich my skin as it loses its elasticity.

I hadn't realised that receding gums was one of the symptoms associated with the perimenopause. For years I have had horrendous trouble with this, though it is gradually improving.

I have started talking openly about my menopause because women so often seem to endure this sometimes-rough journey alone. Why? People talk about puberty, but the menopause is like a forbidden subject. Identifying with other women who are going through it is so important.

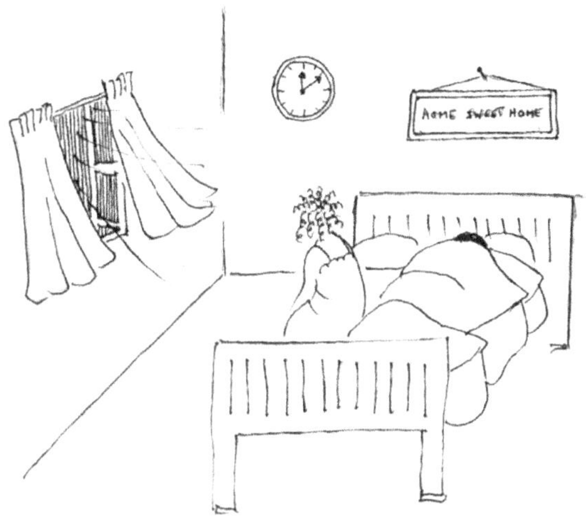

Leigh's story

(a letter from my 59-year-old self to my 49-year-old self)

Dear Leigh,

I realise it's dawning on you that this birthday is not going to be an especially happy one. You're not aware of it, but you've been going through the perimenopause. They didn't talk about this much back then, and even when they did, most people thought it was just women making a fuss – being 'hormonal'. I wish you knew that a decade later, women approaching the menopause would have more of an awareness that things might be peculiar around this time, that they might expect changes in their physical and mental health which would vary for all of them.

Back to 2009… Having been happily married, you will have found yourself wildly attracted to another, less suitable person: drawn to him, even though he was unavailable and significantly less 'safe'. You will have walked away from your marriage and your nice life. You'll have got into trouble at work and been asked to leave. And you won't have been able to understand any of it.

Your 50th year will not be easy. You will struggle badly for money. You will try – and fail – to leave your unavailable man. You will often be alone, frightened and confused, and you will feel like a complete idiot. Please don't feel like that.

You have been through a stage where your hormones, as
you come to the end of your fertile period, have gone
haywire. Rather than petering out gently, yours have
come in fits and starts, leading to spells of wild behaviour,
punctuated by regret and self-recrimination. The words of
others come back to haunt you in the middle of the night:
"You won't make anything of yourself!"; "She never sticks
at anything!"; "Problem sister!"; "Just like your no-good
father!"

At times, I know, it feels as though you have nothing to
live for. But you have *everything* to live for. The next few
years will be tough, but as you go through the gateway
that is your physical menopause, there will be a distinct
change. As the final bursts of oestrogen leave your system,
a new, steely determination will set in. Driven by the
desire to prove you're not a disaster, together with very,
very hard work, you will be able to show yourself, and the
world, that you are worthy of a place on this planet.

At 59, just ten years later, you have achieved an MA in
psychotherapy. You are a clinical supervisor, supporting
counsellors in their clinical work. You run a successful
private practice, and have become a Lecturer in Higher
Education, teaching counselling and psychotherapy. You
will be respected.

And whilst it will be a journey that will not always be easy,
you will find yourself in a happy, healthy relationship with
the same unsuitable man who you 'gave it all up for'.
Despite how it may seem now, your instinct will prove
you correct: he is the person you should be with. The
difficult journey you will share with him will teach you
how to 'do' relationships, will provide you with strength,
and will fill you with joy.

Happy birthday!

Your Future Self x

Sue's story

I was about 45 when I realised something strange was happening to my body. I was experiencing occasional periods of sudden and extreme heat, during which I simply had to cool down. At home, The Battle of the Thermostat commenced. I spent an inordinate amount of time running my wrists under cold water or going to stand outside. In the middle of winter I was out and about with my jacket wide open, or not wearing it at all. My migraines were worse than they'd ever been: I suffered from an almost constant headache.

Eventually, I got fed up enough to see my doctor. I described being hot and bothered, tired and emotional, and jokingly suggested that it might be down to the menopause. I didn't mention the migraines – we talked about those at pretty much every other visit. The doctor did say that my symptoms might be perimenopausal, but I didn't take him seriously and didn't pay the recommended website much attention.

A few months passed and things continued to go downhill. I was in a difficult work situation, which made matters even worse. My anxiety skyrocketed. I couldn't concentrate for more than a few minutes at a time. I struggled to find the easiest words. I wasn't sleeping. I was hot. My joints ached. The migraines were unbearable, and I tended to react to everything very emotionally. I saw my doctor again and requested that my anxiety meds be increased. I also got some great counselling. When I wasn't at work, the anxiety was manageable, but on workdays I was nauseous, tearful and fearful. I gained weight very quickly – all of it around my waist – and my boobs hurt. The migraines continued.

I was only in my mid-forties. I couldn't possibly be hurtling towards the menopause. Surely it was just the stress of being a graduate student, working full-time and having a family?

At this time, I was starting to set up my own business, which focused on midlife. I accidentally fell into a few conversations on social media about the perimenopause: symptoms; treatments; experiences. And the penny finally dropped. I was perimenopausal! That was what was wrong with me! I wasn't going mad. It was real and all those crappy health things…well, they were connected. Talk about a huge relief!

Several months on, I'm doing great. The knowledge and support from other women gave me the confidence to go back and see my doctor and advocate for what I really needed. I don't have it all yet, but I'm getting there. I know what I want to try and where to find the resources to back it up. Not every woman is so lucky. But why didn't I know everything before? Why has there not been education to help women understand what is happening to their bodies? Why do we have to find out the hard way? Why aren't all doctors trained in the menopause?

I still have SO MANY QUESTIONS!

Rachel's story

When early menopause hit at 41, it threw me all over the place. I was devastated, as I'd been trying for a second child. But that was the only reason I found out: a hormone test. I didn't have any symptoms back then. It felt like I'd been catapulted into middle-age and I just wasn't ready for it. So I floundered around, questioning everything about myself: who I was as a suddenly infertile woman, whose only knowledge of menopause was that it happened to older women. I was officially old, and it was all downhill from now on…

But then I realised I was being ageist against myself. I was buying in to all the negative stereotypes about midlife, the menopause and older women. I was accepting society's narrative that menopause is something to be feared, and ageing something to be fought against. I was assuming that beauty was only for the young. I'd bought the anti-ageing products. I thought my value was diminishing as I became less relevant in a world that worships youth and, therefore, fertility.

It took a long time to feel 'me' again and to realise I had everything going for me as a postmenopausal woman. I stopped being anti-ageing. We all age, and trying to fight it is like being anti-night-time! It's going to get you nowhere fast. I learnt a lot about the menopause and how we can transition vibrantly through it. I don't see it as something to be fixed, but as a magnificent transformation in a woman's life to be embraced. Yes, I know it can be hard for some of us. But it is often the negative voices that shout the loudest – and I'm all about redressing the balance.

I reluctantly followed medical advice and went on HRT (the NHS body-identical kind) to protect my bones and heart (because of the menopause coming early and a bone density scan showing borderline osteopenia in my hip). But I was advised that I only needed to be on it until the 'normal' menopause age of 51. So, at 51, I weaned myself off HRT and now manage any symptoms naturally. I occasionally take vaginal oestrogen to help with dryness, but more often than not forget to do this, and lube works pretty well! I've heard that dryness can be more of a problem for women who've not given birth vaginally, which I haven't. That's really the only issue I've had with the menopause transition. Lots of midlife angst, yes, but not necessarily caused directly by the menopause. But I have changed my life to minimise any negative effects.

I now know there are many ways we can naturally help ourselves through menopause. We don't have to be helpless in the face of hot flushes, aches and anxiety. We can take back control and manage our own experience of this important time. There are things we can do and habits we can change or cultivate that will make it all so much more manageable than society or the media would have us believe! HRT doesn't have to be the only solution. I prefer not being on any drug unless it's absolutely necessary.

I believe menopause symptoms are an early warning that there may be things about our lives we need to change, if we want long-term health. I also believe menopause can highlight and exacerbate existing physical or psychological issues, rather than necessarily cause them. I think it often gets a bad rap and is very easy to blame. I like to see it as the canary in the coal mine.

My research made me realise I needed to change my lifestyle to live well. I needed to reduce my stress (which

I'm sure contributed to menopause coming early) and look after myself much better. I upped my exercise (particularly running and yoga) and sorted out my diet, eating more organically (including plenty of natural phytoestrogens) and trying to limit alcohol and sugar (often unsuccessfully, but they sure do cause hot flushes!). I cut out caffeine, started to practise meditation to manage stress and anxiety, tried to eliminate toxins in cleaning and cosmetic products (which can mess with our hormones) and got proactive about what I wanted for my next chapter, rather than doing what I'd always done.

The menopause was a timestamp for me, and it spurred me to action. It's when I embarked on my mission: to change all that bollocks that had gripped me so acutely when I got the early menopause diagnosis. I don't want women to fear the menopause: it's a natural rite of passage – and a glorious one at that. I want them to embrace this time and feel the power that comes with age and confidence. It's not the end, but an exciting new beginning. We've been working with our wombs all our lives. I don't believe the menopause is the time to start fighting them.

Bizarrely, I have become known for talking about the menopause, and women make a beeline for me at events to chat about this very topic! I could never have forecast that for myself! But I'm all about ending the taboo.

So an early menopause was the trigger for my own journey of self-discovery and reinvention – and also for my new life as an entrepreneur! It's been a real gift. My priorities have shifted, and I want real purpose in my life now. I'm already at least halfway through, but if I consider what I achieved between 20 and 50, I see no reason why I can't achieve just as much between 50 and 80. That's my plan, anyhow!

I believe that if we have our health and look after ourselves (and I mean *really* look after ourselves), we get better with age, not worse (apart from a hopefully-short period of decline at the end of life). I did my first half-marathon at 50, my first modelling gig at 51 and I've built three websites since I turned 49. The end of our fertility can be an incredibly fertile time, and we must invest in it. We are off the Oestrogen Rollercoaster and are calmer, often more creative, more confident and certainly more powerful. I hope you'll join me in stepping up, not back!

Lauraine's story

13th January 2015 was to be a life-changing day for me. I was due to have a hysterectomy with removal of my ovaries, an operation which would end years of misery and uncertainty caused by severe endometriosis and a suspect mass.

The prospect of losing my ovaries worried me. The more I read, the more I realised that these vital organs play a small but significant part long after menopause. My consultant reassured me that I wouldn't notice any difference as mine were so diseased they probably weren't working anyway. Plus, there was the suspect mass they needed to get out.

The loss of my ovaries turned out to be the least of my worries. As a result of severe endometriosis and bowel disease, my uterus, ovaries and all things gynaecological had fused to my bowel, tricking all the experts into thinking it might be something sinister. This mass had been sitting there patiently for many years, until the surgeon's knife cut into it and released the sleeping dragon…

Two days after the surgery I felt like death. I was unable to get out of bed and the thought of food made me wretch. I was eventually persuaded to stand up and walk around the bed. After a few seconds, I felt something warm and sticky running down my leg. I looked down to see a green puddle on the floor. It seemed to be coming from my vagina. My bowel had perforated. At that moment my life changed forever. I was in hospital for a very traumatic three months, being vein-fed with the possibility of never eating or drinking again. The hospital was a hundred miles away from home, and life as I knew it crumbled.

I left hospital having developed an enterocutaneous fistula, which meant I had a connection between my small bowel and skin which spewed out poo day and night. I ended up with three stoma bags, a damaged bladder, gallbladder issues, constant pain and a myriad of other problems. I was a broken wreck – and worse was to come. Trying to come to terms with my new normal was difficult, to say the least. I couldn't eat normally, could barely move without pain or some ominous-looking fluid coming from my lady-bits, and was also having to deal with the horrors of three stoma bags, which leaked every single day. On top of this, I had now been plunged into a surgical menopause, which completed my feelings of total wipe-out.

However, because I had such a serious physical illness (an enterocutaneous fistula is classified as being a surgical catastrophe), nobody seemed to appreciate the effect the menopause was having on me. The night sweats, crushing depression, anxiety, sadness, irritability and feelings of worthlessness were all 'normalised' in the light of what I had been through. After all, I was "lucky to be alive". Plus, of course, I didn't know what was causing what. Was it the menopause creating all these problems or the fact that I'd lost one of life's greatest gifts – my health? It was hard to tell, but I definitely sensed that the loss of my ovaries was adding to my despair. I missed 'me'. The simplicity of my old life had gone.

My husband wrote: "I miss my wife – the funny, capable, confident, feisty woman I married. Yes, she'd had more than her fair share of health issues all our married life, but nothing like this. A perforated bowel and all that entails, plus the ravages of the menopause, would have been too much for many, and indeed many times I thought I WOULD lose her, her depression was so unrelenting. No one ever listened though – the menopause wasn't even considered. She was told she'd get used to it, that she should up the antidepressants, or get some counselling. She once asked me how I'd feel if someone had ripped my testicles off and damaged my bowel in the process. I couldn't answer, but it made me focus on the enormity of what had happened to her. I'm just glad men don't go through the menopause. I find it difficult to find the right words to console her: it has almost broken us after forty years together."

Four years later

I am now 58 and have never recovered, either physically or mentally, from the fall-out of that fateful decision to have a hysterectomy. It plunged me and my family into hell. I still have the stoma bags and chronic ill-health – and dealing with the menopause on top of this has been soul-destroying. The anxiety is crippling, my self-esteem rock-bottom. I feel worthless, invisible and irrelevant. My relationship with my husband has been severely affected, with intimacy a distant memory.

I feel mutilated by the hysterectomy, not just because of the bowel perforation that resulted from it, but different as a woman as well. I feel almost bereaved at my loss of femininity. I feel old and unattractive. I have asked about HRT but have been told it's a bad idea: I am "too old" and it would "reignite the endometriosis". Apparently, I will "get used to it".

The gynaecologist who performed the hysterectomy did write to my GP to say that he wasn't opposed to me trying HRT. At last I felt that here was some recognition of the problems the menopause had brought me, but when I discussed it with the GP, he completely discouraged me and said it might cause more problems and that he didn't want to be the one "to add more spice to the mix". I felt as though I'd been well and truly sent out into the wilderness.

The future

I'm trying to be kinder to myself. I'm learning to say no and put myself first occasionally. I meditate when it all gets too much. I make damned sure I get my hair done or my nails painted when I feel up to it. Having several invisible conditions when you look reasonably OK but feel like a train wreck is difficult, as empathy is sometimes in short supply. I now have two beautiful granddaughters who bring me so much joy and happiness. I also have my 10-year-old nephews who I love dearly and are a big part of my life. I'm trying to enjoy the many good things and make every day count. I've lost too much as it is. I'm lucky to be surrounded by family and friends who look out for me as I look out for them. I muddle through as best I can.

The effects of my menopause made a dreadful situation almost impossible to deal with. I'm still hopeful for brighter days, when the crippling symptoms ease and I can cope better with everything else. I'd always been told that the menopause would be my panacea, because the endometriosis would improve. But instead it has been the worst time of my life and certainly not 'The Change' I was hoping for.

Margaret's story

I'm a pessimist. When I was approaching the age when I could expect to begin 'The Change', I read a lot of books about the subject, collecting advice.

It turned out to be unnecessary. The menopause had little effect on me. I didn't have hot flushes, just warm ones – and they never lasted long. I was more tired than usual, but then I did lead a very busy life. I was moodier, too – or so my husband said! My periods became lighter (although they were never heavy). One day they stopped, then after a while started again, and a few months later stopped altogether.

I've no idea why I had such an easy time of it. Many of my friends didn't.

Ali's story

(or *I Hate My Reproductive System: Let Me Count the Ways* –
with apologies to Ray Davies)

Thank you for the pain,

The endless days and days of pain you gave me.

It got me out of Games

But netball might have been preferred in hindsight.

Nights when I couldn't sleep all night,

Days when I couldn't stand upright,

You made me puke

And cost me loads and loads and loads of money.

All sorts of pads, tampons and different kinds of
analgesics,

To no avail…

Sitting by a fan

And turning pink and red and puce and purple.

I can't rip off my clothes

But let me tell you now,

I really want to.

Hot flushes don't sound all that bad

Until you've had them, then you know

How they creep up

At inconvenient moments

And make you look

As though you've started melting.

It's pretty grim…

Thank you for the day

When both my ovaries expired entirely.

Let joy be unconfined

And pads with wings be just consigned to memory.

No more ripping out my pubes,

No more dashing to the loo.

You took my life

And now I'm happy that you're going to leave me.

But it's alright.

I'm not that scared of HRT, believe me.

But no libido…

Thank you for the bleed

That happened twelve months after my last period.

The GP frowned

And said, "It's possible that could be cancer."

Thankfully tests were negative,

Internal ultrasound was clear,

There's nothing like

A pokey stick

To reassure you that your bits are normal,

If somewhat wizened…

Katie's story

I was 43 when I knew I didn't feel quite 'right'.

I can't put my finger on what exactly was wrong. I just know that I was heading home from the school-run and felt empty, numb and slow. It was as if I was walking through a fog, through thick treacle, slightly disconnected. I felt low, tired, anxious and not sure what my purpose was in life, now that my youngest had finally started going to school all day.

I put it down to being the mum of four kids, juggling family and home-life with work.

But things got progressively worse. I didn't have the energy to cook a meal, tidy the house, make decisions. I no longer enjoying socialising. I stopped finding things funny. I comfort-ate to try and 'feel' something, but this just made me gain tonnes of weight, which in turn made me very self-conscious, and I became a hermit who never wanted to go out, see people, or even phone anyone.

I went to the doctor – a young man who looked not much older than my son – and asked what this mixed bag of symptoms could mean. After about five minutes, he sent me on my way with a prescription for antidepressants.

A month later I felt no different. In fact, I felt worse. I was numb: getting on with life but not living. I started to forget words at meetings, couldn't remember where I'd left things and became convinced that I was suffering from early-onset dementia. I was constantly teary, which was very embarrassing, and felt ashamed of the woman I had become.

At my next visit to the doctor's, the GP said I was probably stressed from juggling so many different things, and suggested I give up work for a while. I took his advice, left my job and gave myself some time off, determined to try and take things a bit easier. But then the heavy periods began. Little did I know, but I was becoming seriously anaemic, which caused heart palpitations and made me sleep for most of the day. Convinced I was suffering from ME, or having a heart attack, I trotted off for a third trip to the GP. This time he sent me off for heart tests. Nothing showed up.

Then the backache kicked in. The doctor said I was just overweight and should take up Pilates. He added that it was probably all in my mind and humiliated me by asking if I wanted to see a psychiatrist. I felt utter despair. Was I going mad? Here I was, a happily married woman with four fantastic kids, living in a lovely house, surrounded by family and friends. What was wrong with me? Why couldn't I enjoy life? Where had I gone? And how could I get 'me' back?

For four years I was tested for everything under the sun – and made to feel like I was losing my mind. It was only then that my father, who is a breast cancer professor, suggested that it might be hormone-related, and that I should see a gynaecologist who specialised in hormones.

After giving me a blood test, and taking a full history of my symptoms, the gynaecologist uttered just one word: PERIMENOPAUSE. She explained that my oestrogen levels were on the floor and that they were the *entire* reason I was feeling all these things. She reassured me that nothing was wrong with me, suggested I had a coil fitted to stop the bleeding, and told me I'd feel like a new woman after a month on HRT.

And she was right. Four weeks later, my mood had lifted significantly, my energy levels had peaked, my memory had returned, I could think clearly and make normal decisions, the anxiety and palpitations had stopped, and I suddenly realised I was happy and really enjoying my life again. It was the first time in years that I could remember laughing and 'feeling'. My husband said he had got his wife back.

That evening, as I cried my eyes out with relief, I turned to Facebook to see if anyone else could relate to my years of perimenopausal hell. All the women's groups I could find were for mums with young babies, comparing notes on nappy-rash and buggies. So I decided to set up my own group. I wanted it to feel like an online coffee shop for mid-life women, since I've always found chatting with a friend over a latte is the solution to most of life's problems.

To my utter surprise, within twenty-four hours of setting up the group, I had two thousand members. In two days, that had doubled. And so The Latte Lounge (Top Tips for Women over 40) was created. Today, after three years, we have over sixteen thousand women across sixty-nine countries onboard. I have since established a website (www.lattelounge.co), put together a medical advisory committee and assembled more than thirty contributors to help support women in all areas of mid-life, so that no one ever needs to feel alone, confused, lost, or like they're going mad. I am also using the platform to raise money and awareness for The Eve Appeal, the UK's gynaecological cancer prevention and early diagnosis research charity.

Doctors need better training to understand and spot symptoms of the perimenopause, and women need to be educated from an early age about it, too. After all, when it hit me, I wasn't having hot flushes and still had periods. But in the ten years before menopause, as oestrogen levels start to drop, women can experience symptoms that are the same as (or even worse than) those experienced around menopause itself.

I feel angry that I lost four precious years of my life, and I want my forum to be the go-to place for all things mid-life, so that we can be a force for good. We can campaign for better education and awareness, provide up-to-date, evidence-based information, and support and signpost women correctly so they get the help they need, when they need it.

Helen's story

I entered surgical menopause at 41. That makes it sound like a grand entrance into the New Year's Eve Ball at the Imperial Palace in Vienna. But it was more a falling-off-the-edge-of-a-cliff, and it took seemingly forever to hit the ground. And the moment of impact wasn't pretty.

I spent three years in freefall before advocating for myself – or rather my husband advocating for me – and insisting that I be offered HRT. Within a fortnight of starting it, my stiff, achy joints disappeared, and I experienced episodes of deep, restorative sleep.

However, during those three years I had a breakdown, resigned from a job that I loved dearly, had a relapse in the depression that I had been managing well for two decades, and got to a point where I went to bed each night hoping that I would not wake up.

My situation was compounded by the fact that I had always struggled with any form of interpersonal engagement, which made explaining to my GP how I felt extremely challenging. What was more, I couldn't cope with even the slightest change in my highly regimented daily routine – I needed sameness, day in, day out. I was one confused, frustrated and desperate woman.

Menopause is referred to as 'The Change' for a reason. It brings on a whole heap of changes, and I found these impossible to manage. To cut a long story short, at the age of 46 I was identified as being on the autistic spectrum. Life started to make sense.

So, in a way, I have a lot to thank my surgical menopause for. Without it, I probably wouldn't have had a breakdown and might never have known that many of the struggles I had growing up were largely due to my autism. In that sense, it was a blessing.

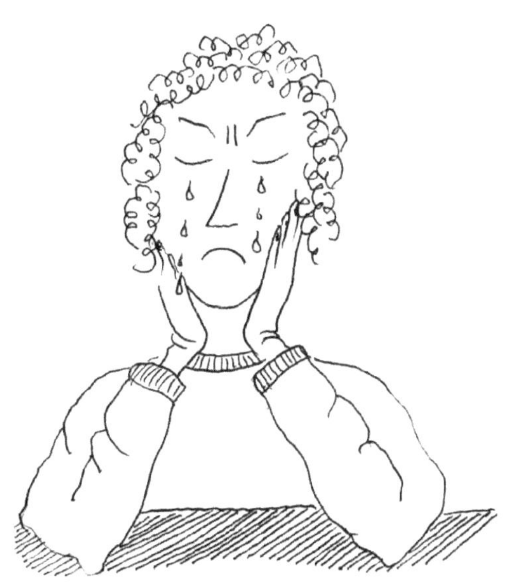

Michele's story

There's a lot of secrecy surrounding the menopause. Many women really suffer with it but are scared to talk about it for fear of condemnation from those of their sisters who have an easier time and think they're drama queens. Have a look at the Menopause Matters forum to get a feel for the problems the menopause can cause and the struggles many women have finding suitable HRT (if this is the route they have chosen).

The ignorance and lack of understanding from GPs is considerable. Many cling to outdated beliefs and want us out of their surgeries as fast as possible with a prescription for antidepressants. A fair number of us are forced to pay for private treatment. There are also a lot of snake-oil salesmen out there, willing to take money for ineffective and unregulated treatments. Employers are not at all sympathetic and too many women are forced to give up work.

Of course, not all women struggle as badly as the 25% of the female population who are worst affected. You'll probably have guessed by now that I am one of that 25%: a bright, educated professional who had to give up work at 56 after four years of struggling to cope. I'm now 59, and although I'm in a better place, I'm a shadow of my former self. I get on with it, but wish I'd known what can happen if you're unlucky enough to have a difficult menopause. It's a country-mile away from the low moods and hot flushes we've all been led to expect, and I was totally upended by it. More people are talking about it now and things are definitely improving, but it's still a subject surrounded by secrecy and shame.

I'm in a very fortunate position. I have an understanding husband and a lovely life, but I wish I could enjoy it more. I don't find the menopause at all empowering. Quite the opposite. The more books there are on what it's really like, the better. It might make women realise that they're not losing their minds. Or that there's not something seriously wrong with them. Here's my story…

I went to my GP when I was 52 and still having monthly periods. I was a bit of a mess and holding down a stressful job with lots of travelling. The GP said, "Yep, I get it, we'll start you on oestrogen and give you a Mirena coil." She was great.

However, one of her colleagues disagreed and basically told me to get my big girl pants on and go away. I then spent eighteen months trying every herbal remedy to no avail, rapidly going downhill mentally (total nut-job, rages, anger, crying, shouting) and physically (tummy problems, joint and muscle pains, brain fog, exhaustion, insomnia, still having periods with flooding, bad flushes, terrible hair and skin, palpitations, panic attacks). At times, I thought I was dying.

Another doctor told me that I was depressed and that antidepressants would help stabilise my moods. But I hallucinated on them and was told to stop taking them immediately. A locum GP agreed to start me on HRT if I could explain the risks to her and if I understood that my decision to go on it was entirely mine. I was 54 and still in perimenopause. It took multiple visits to finally get a prescription. I spent the next year taking HRT, which made me feel significantly worse. I felt as if I was being poisoned and my mental state deteriorated. There are three flights of stairs in our house and at times I could only crawl up the last flight. I hardly left the house for ten months and sank into a deep depression.

Eventually, I went down the private route, and thankfully my current doctor listens to me and understands me. I was given body-identical oestrogen and progesterone, and after some tweaking of my prescription (I went from gel to patches), I began to feel much better. Having said that, the progesterone causes me some problems, so I may try to come off it…

Throughout all this, I had various spells off work, but concessions were never made, and so I negotiated a settlement to leave. The stress of the job wasn't helping my mental health. I'm more settled these days – but somehow, sadly, I've lost my vibrancy and sense of identity. At the risk of sounding dramatic, I've lost 'me'.

Something has gone and I'm not sure it will ever come back...

Greta's story

When you google 'menopause symptoms' you get 'About 92,700,000 results (0.56 seconds)'. Ninety-two million, seven hundred thousand. That's a lot of research (and there are some gems of very good advice amongst the depressing lists of symptoms) but it's the personal stories that have helped me the most, so I offer you my own ongoing story in three short acts in the hope that it might help you.

Act 1: 1986. Me and my mum

My mum died when she was 42, at the same time as she was going through the menopause. She started early, at 40. I was 18 and my parents had recently divorced. Mum described herself as "sad and mad" and was prescribed antidepressants by her sixty-something male GP who "never had the time to listen". The pills made a lethal cocktail when mixed with the gin and fortified wine she was downing in increasing amounts in a bid to escape from this new version of herself. She did escape. She didn't die of the menopause, but the effects of it exacerbated a number of complex problems. Everyone stopped listening to her because a menopausal alcoholic is not someone anybody wants to spend time with. And she knew it. I was doing my A levels and trying to keep a sense of normality, both for her and for me.

After she died, I learnt about the symptoms and effects of the menopause and vowed that when my turn came, I'd damn well be ready for it. I felt sure that the medical world would have made huge inroads into understanding it better by then and that by the time I was in my late forties/early fifties, the world would be ready for me and my heated mood-swings.

Act 2: 2012. Me and my partner

I met someone when I was 44. My marriage had broken down and this was a new start. A couple of months later the hot flushes began. The deep unease and sadness I had been feeling (which had been masked by the chemical and emotional rush of a new relationship) started to add up to the menopause. The worst bit was the creeping realisation that this new version of me was battling with the woman I wanted my new partner to know: the 'old' me, the one he said he had fallen in love with at first sight. But that woman was dripping away… My hair was coming out in handfuls, I itched my ears red-raw and everything ached. I couldn't walk downhill without sharp pain in my knees. Or uphill, come to that. I felt leaden, unattractive, angry and I could practically feel my bones crumbling inside my ever-thinning skin.

My partner insisted that he couldn't see any of this. He was kind and loving, but I pushed him away. I didn't want him to see me like this and became convinced that he would find someone new in a matter of weeks – or even days. Why would he still want me when he could be with someone young, taut and vibrant? Someone fertile? He had no children and was younger than me. He still had choices and I had none. At least, that's how it felt.

He told me none of this mattered, but I couldn't bear the heat of him next to me in bed. You know that part of a new relationship where you want the very bones of the person beside you, day and night? Well, that had gone. Why would he stay? I exhausted him with my negativity, assuring him, "I'm normally so positive, such an optimist, with shiny hair and glowing skin, honest!" – and he told me over and over that he loved me. Damn his positivity!

I was determined not to go to my GP, but after two years, feeling utterly exhausted, I went. She was a young woman, and heavily pregnant. I don't think she could help it, but she looked at me through her glow as if I was something to be got rid of as soon as possible before I contaminated both her and her room with my rinsed-out desperation. She asked me what I wanted. I said I didn't know: just some relief. After googling some stuff in front of me, she told me that HRT was not an option because I suffered from migraines. She suggested I breathe through it. I thought I was going to scream but smiled instead and went home.

I returned to her a year later, on my knees, and she – now harried and with her breasts leaking – wrote me out a prescription for HRT without even asking what I wanted. I googled what she'd given me when I got home and binned it.

Act 3: 2019. Me

The tide is now turning, but very slowly. Every thread about the menopause follows a similar pattern, with women feeling hopeless, helpless and disenfranchised by their dramatically-changing bodies. I've stopped googling these threads now, but knowledge has become both my armour and my remedy. I know my body again, inside and out. I know this new me. Trial and error have led me to find things that really help me: urtica (nettle tincture) for itchy skin and hot flushes (and with the added bonus of giving me shiny hair); ashwagandha for low moods and adrenal function; minerals and vitamins for bones, eyesight and a clear head; glucosamine and krill oil for my joints; exercise; seeing friends; having a focus outside work (I've started to paint and love it); going to bed earlier when I can; cotton sheets. Oh, and reading. Philosophy has really helped: learning that I can influence how I react to events, that there are some things within my control. All this helps, and I feel empowered by working it out on my own.

The flushes have lessened over the years and I feel mentally stronger than I have ever done (counselling is helping) and physically good again. The menopause is a huge thing, and I think about my mum every day and wish she'd been given urtica instead of antidepressants and had someone to talk to instead of putting-up and shutting-up. But she wasn't – and she didn't.

Every single woman who goes through the menopause experiences it differently, and each deserves to be listened to. IT IS SO IMPORTANT.

Epilogue

The menopause is still largely ignored and treated as 'other' by the medical profession (certainly by the professionals I've come across). I know if it happened to men, too, there would be much more money ploughed into trying to understand (and treat) it better. I know this because men have told me that once they have direct experience of the menopause (through the suffering of partners, mothers, friends, sisters etc.), they feel pretty damn strongly about it. In the past, women scarcely mentioned it, leaving their sons to assume it wasn't a problem and their daughters completely unprepared for what was coming. And as it's the sons who still largely run the world, very little has been done: if their mothers put up with it, then why can't their wives and partners?

Well, I have two sons and have brought them up knowing what it means to go through the menopause. We are doing no one any favours when we hide the reality of what 50% of the population have to go through. So let's continue the heated debate (pun fully intended).

Karen C's story

I had a hysterectomy at 35 – but wasn't plunged into an early menopause as I kept my ovaries. It wasn't until I was about 48 that I started to develop symptoms. To begin with, I just noticed the occasional hot flush, but it wasn't long before these – and the night sweats that accompanied them – became debilitating. I really need my sleep to function, and my daily routine was affected because I was constantly tired.

I didn't want to go down the HRT route, preferring instead to try a more natural approach. I experimented with black cohosh and soy vitamins, but neither seemed to work for me. I found that taking sage tablets helped a little and discovered that spicy foods and alcohol made my hot flushes worse and more frequent.

I worried about getting hot flushes when out with friends: it's not very helpful when people point out that your face is bright red! The embarrassment seemed to increase the intensity and duration of the flushes, though I refused to let them stop me having a social life.

Itchy skin was an unexpected and incredibly irritating symptom, and brain fog was another daily occurrence. I often found I put the teapot in the fridge and the milk in the cupboard! There was one occasion when I was making a Bolognese sauce and suddenly thought to myself, "I haven't put the kidney beans in!" I'd switched to thinking I was making a chilli… Once I'd added the beans to my sauce, I got the pasta out and realised I was making chilli after all! I served it up to my husband who said it was still lovely, so I decided I'd invented a new dish and called it Bolognelli! It's now a (somewhat odd) family favourite, so I guess there are some benefits to having brain fog after all!

During my quest to discover more natural remedies, my son started training in Reflexology. I found this technique so relaxing, and very effective in helping me sleep. I was even more thrilled when his training led him to develop a cream with a blend of essential oils in it to help with my hot flushes and night sweats, which he has since launched and called Menomagic. It helps with both my sleep and my itchy skin.

Now, at 59, I'm still experiencing some symptoms, and looking forward to the day when it's all over – but I'm determined to laugh through whatever the menopause throws at me. Laughter is one of the best remedies for any frustration in life!

Amber's story

I read the first volume of *The Menopause Monologues* quickly and immediately passed it on to my husband. It was especially timely given that I'd been on my own menopause journey for the previous few months…or maybe years.

Following an intense and traumatic couple of weeks earlier this year, my hot flushes started with a bang; I went from experiencing zero to ten or twenty a day. At first, I thought I was coming down with a temperature, but realisation soon dawned. This must be it…

I was 44 and had been period-free since my Mirena coil was fitted seven years before. I was also in the middle of a consultation process to remove a ten-centimetre ovarian cyst. When I told the gynaecologist about these hot flushes, he suggested that if my ovaries had stopped working, they could be removed at the same time (to prevent ovarian cancer), and so he ran a test for FSH levels. This checks for the hormone which stimulates the ovaries to release eggs and should apparently be under 30 if you are fertile and over 30 if you are menopausal. Mine came back at 115…

This news, coupled with the general stress I was under, left me feeling completely overwhelmed. I needed to decide what to do about these 'useless' ovaries of mine and on top of this was wrestling with how on earth I could possibly be postmenopausal (as the gynae was intimating) when the hot flushes were the first symptom I had experienced.

I am normally quite pragmatic and measured, but all this really unsettled me. I felt like my body was letting me down. I googled relentlessly. Could the coil have masked what was going on? Could the cyst be causing the problems? What would be the outcome of removing my ovaries? But I struggled to get concrete answers.

I was also researching menopausal symptoms – and came to realise that the previous three years had been clouded by anxiety, a sense of impending doom, even worse sleep than normal (I have been a terrible insomniac since my early twenties), headaches, aching joints, general lethargy, panic attacks and palpitations.

I'm usually a glass-half-full person and had put all these symptoms down to the stress of work and bringing up teenagers. I'd certainly not thought about combining them to point to a single cause.

So, I was menopausal then? It felt enormously shocking to me. And I still needed to decide what to do about those shrivelled ovaries.

I asked for another FSH test. This one came back at 55, and I began to wonder how much the stress I'd been under had impacted my hormones. So I decided to proceed with the cyst removal but hang on to the ovaries: I didn't want to risk plunging myself into a sudden 'menopausal cloud' if I was still producing enough oestrogen after all. A week or two before the operation my hot flushes stopped as quickly as they had started.

After I recovered from the operation, I started to feel like a new person: lighter, brighter – much more my positive self. Had the cyst caused my symptoms? I asked my GP for a final FSH test, still labouring under this feeling that my body was impersonating someone else. It came back at 28. One last twist to the story: I found a breast lump in June. It turned out to be a benign cyst, but the (very sympathetic) breast consultant told me that hormonal swings can often cause these.

A few months on, I'm not feeling quite so light and bright, but I'm definitely no longer suffering from the levels of anxiety, palpitations, hot flushes, poor sleep (for me) and low energy that I was before. I would really like a proper explanation for what I've been through – and am frustrated by the lack of it. Whilst reading the first volume of *The Menopause Monologues*, I noted that for some people symptoms started and then disappeared for a while, so maybe that's where I am. I also wonder a lot about stress and the impact that has on one physically.

But at least now I feel much more prepared for when it all comes back. And when it does, I won't put up with feeling low, anxious, exhausted and achy, because I don't want to waste precious time experiencing my life through a miserable, grey fog.

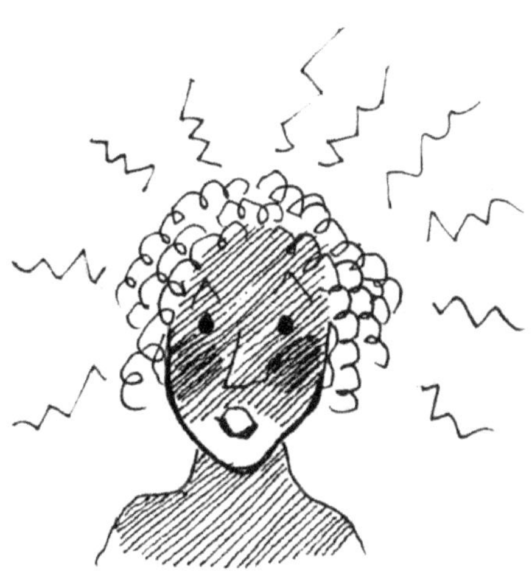

Moya's story

Precisely how or when I transitioned from sex kitten to Bagpuss remains a mystery. I now find myself in the privileged position of having to shave only as far as the knee – and sometimes just the shin will suffice. I'm certainly not overjoyed at the realisation that I am now part of a nation that can live in a nice static home. I'm no fashion guru either and will not be that plus-size model setting a trend for support socks on flights anytime soon. (My croc addiction should doubly ensure this.) I am done with waistbands that cut, parting flesh like a knife: it's elastication all the way to the funeral parlour for me.

Hormones and the menopause: uninspiring subjects, but their impact remains unheeded. Compassion (and also consideration) for your female counterparts is all I ask. Having just turned 53 – and fourteen months period-free – I sit here with everything crossed, hoping that I really am through it and emerging from that epic chapter of life.

From birth, hormones exist, unseen and simmering in the carcass of an innocent framework. Puberty hits and the simmering increases, the imposters often stripping us of the knowledge of who we are. We have no choice but to offer them the residence they require.

A few years may pass until our bodies become warm havens for new life. The imposters return from their hibernation, determined to complete their task. Anxiously, we accept their existence, reassured by their role in preparing our bodies to deliver that new life.

Things remain unsettled. We acknowledge their presence, always aware that our relationship with them is rocky.

Years go by until they revisit, but now they take up unrestricted residence. It's the Perimenopausal Torture Tour. The dormant volcano awakens; we are left stunned, helpless, and soaked in their residue.

My mind has raced as if it is band-searching a radio. I hold the arrival of testosterone fully responsible for the farting and overnight emergence of unfathomably long, rogue hairs. Thankfully, I have so far eluded the 'All the kids have gone, let's get a dog!' scenario.

The hormones' ebbing is too slow. Imagined encores delay their eventual departure. Our fertile bodies remain a battlefield until we can lay down our arms and venture out into the barren no-man's-land, where at last they take flight. Their day is done.

My bra is moulded to me beautifully, chewing-gum grey and comfortable; it's taken some time to get it to this point. Rest assured: I have no intention of burning it.

I'm celebrating on this sunny day – no longer a slave. I'm feeling quite brave, so I'll wear my white jeans without fear (elasticated waistband 100% guaranteed)!

Clare J's story

"Your blood test results have come back and you're well into menopause. In fact, you're well into *premature* menopause!"

Boom! The word MENOPAUSE explodes in my ears. The floor falls from beneath me. What did the GP just say? I'm 42 – she can't be right! The words go round and round inside my head. The doctor is wearing a sad face. "Don't worry," she continues. "We slapped HRT patches on my mum when she wasn't looking. She was a right bitch. You're young and we need to get the most out of your body. There's a risk of osteoporosis. But there are also risks associated with taking HRT so young – cancer, stroke etc. You can only take it for two years…"

On and on she goes, but I'm still trying to process the first line of the conversation. I'm a Holistic therapist and up till now I've managed my health with herbal medicine, diet, meditation and exercise. But I am feeling vulnerable and she has terrified me – and I find myself leaving with a prescription for HRT.

On autopilot I go to the pharmacy and pay nearly £20; apparently, I need both types of hormones because I'm still menstruating (although irregularly). And this will be something I have to do monthly. I go home and cry…

Thinking back, my menopause began when I was 35. I gave birth to my son in the September of that year and already had a 3-year-old. A couple of months later, my periods restarted and I bled heavily. My health visitor reassured me that after having a second child the womb stretches further than it does with your firstborn, so has a larger surface area from which to bleed when periods return. But the bleeding became harder and harder to manage. I was often soaking through pads within the hour. I felt exhausted and out-of-breath and was diagnosed as being severely anaemic. I took iron and adjusted my diet to eat iron-rich foods, but things didn't improve. I know now that I was suffering from flooding, a symptom common to the perimenopause, but back then I was oblivious.

Winter came. I started waking in the night, drenched in sweat. It was the year swine flu broke out, and I was convinced I was ill. I was wiped out, my immune system was low, and I just kept telling myself I had a virus. It still didn't enter my head that this was the perimenopause. I thought it happened much later. I returned to work when my son turned twelve months and then the stress really kicked in. I was juggling a stressful career, working with children in the care system, and caring for my own two little ones. I felt isolated, ill and completely exhausted. Some days I would get into work without remembering the thirty-minute drive to get there. My son didn't sleep through until he was 3, so on top of everything else I was sleep-deprived. In six weeks, I lost two stone – and my relationship with my partner deteriorated. I felt he didn't understand the demands I was managing. If the children were ill, it was always me who had to take the time off work. I was taken to task over this at work after both my children had chicken pox within two weeks of each other…and that was when things got really difficult.

By the age of 37, I noticed that my periods were becoming erratic. Sometimes I'd have gaps of 45 days between them, sometimes just 18. Because the bleeding was still heavy, I was advised to try the coil, and bled every day for six months with cramping pains. I had it removed and my GP suggested I have a thermal ablation, as the only option after that was a hysterectomy and there was no way I wanted to go down that route. So I had the ablation. My periods stopped for a few months and then came back, but lighter this time.

I was still getting night sweats and constantly felt hot when I was at work. I was experiencing pain every other month around ovulation. Something didn't feel right and now my pelvic floor felt compromised, too. I was diagnosed with an ovarian cyst and a Level 1 prolapse.

My periods became more irregular. I remember feeling like a boat adrift at sea. My menstrual cycle had always been a solid anchor for me – I could set my energy, food cravings, sleep pattern and emotions by where I was up to in my cycle – but now this had vanished. I didn't know what was going on.

I was 42, and the past five years had been seriously rough. I just wanted to be left alone. I didn't want to care for anybody else. I would cry for no reason. Some days I would dream of taking off on an adventure all by myself – but then the guilt would set in. There were days when I wanted to lie in bed all day and sleep, but this wasn't an option. My career didn't feel fulfilling anymore and I took redundancy against my partner's wishes. I went back to college and retrained as a Holistic therapist.

Then the migraines started (another classic symptom of the perimenopause). I returned to my GP and a referral was made for an MRI scan, but it was here that she questioned me about my menstrual cycle and decided to check my hormone levels. The MRI scan showed nothing, but when my blood test results came back, I was asked to make another appointment.

And that was when I got the news. Premature menopause. Boom!

I'm now nearly 47 and in the past five years have made it my mission to find out about the menopause. I have read numerous books, attended many workshops and am currently training to be a Menopause Specialist. Alongside two dear friends, I set up a Menopause Café locally. Why? Because the one lesson being menopausal taught me is that it can be very isolating. Each woman's experience is unique to her and there is still a lot of shame around the subject. Our society values youth and beauty, so women perhaps understandably find it hard to talk about their menopausal health – vaginal dryness, prolapses, libido, hairiness, thinning hair, sore breasts, hot flushes, migraines, anxiety and so on – but we provide them with a safe space, and everyone is welcome.

I regularly see women at my practice and support them through their menopause journey, signposting them to information, recommending books and making them aware of everything that is out there to assist them. I love this quote by Michelle Obama: "I think it's the worst thing that we do to each other as women, not share the truth about our bodies and how they work." This is exactly why I set up my local Menopause Café: to share knowledge and resources, and remove the shame, guilt and fear so that every woman feels supported.

I'm in a great place now. I discovered Arvigo therapy, which rectified my prolapse and helped me nurture and connect with my womb. I look after myself, meditate regularly and rarely have sugar. I have cut out dairy and gluten and eat a healthy, balanced diet. I'm on a voyage of discovery about who I am and what I want, because somewhere in the process of settling down and having a family, I lost sight of my desires, hopes and dreams. I'm delving into the shadows, and confronting my past, my conditioning, my values and my beliefs. It's messy and sometimes hard, but every time I attend a workshop and do the work, another layer lifts and I see things as they truly are.

Menopause is likened to labour pains: birthing your true self is never easy but the end result is miraculous. I'm looking forward to stepping into my Wise Woman stage and donning my Crone crown.

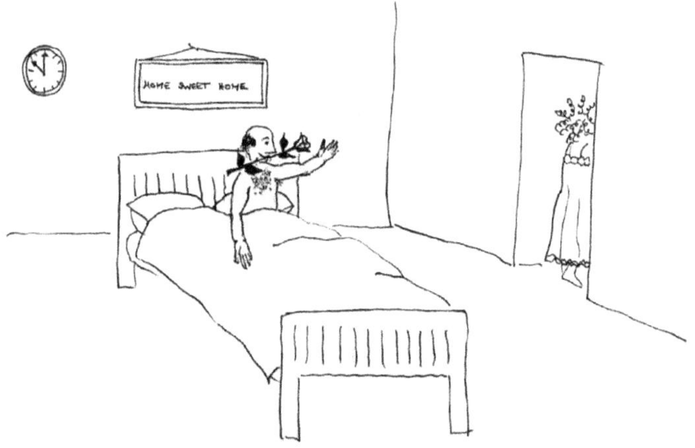

Juliet's story

These days I like to introduce myself as "Juliet: 54 years young, and loving life!" There's no word in Japanese for menopause: they talk instead about being re-energised, about having a "Second Spring", so I'll go with that one, too!

However, it hasn't always been this way…

At around the age of 45, I started to experience hot flushes (probably thirty a day – and burning hot), broken sleep (though I've never slept very well anyway), night sweats and brain fog. I couldn't remember my team's names at work and had to buy two of every top so I could change at lunchtime.

Then I noticed more symptoms: my hands often shook, and I felt dizzy. I arranged to see my GP, who advised a blood test to measure my hormone levels, but over the next eighteen months all the tests came back normal.

However, I knew that something wasn't right. You know your own body and mind, don't you?

I was in a management role, leading a team in HR, and had always been known as someone who would get things done on time and on budget. I delivered presentations, collaborated with senior stakeholders and colleagues, delivered initiatives with fabulous feedback, and loved my work in Leadership and Development. But all this started to change. I was losing my confidence, experiencing panic attacks and heart palpitations, and becoming seriously anxious over things that had never bothered me before.

I would be in tears during most of my commute. I had a fantastic life, a gorgeous husband, an adorable son, an amazing job, a great line-manager and wonderful friends. And yet I felt trapped in a body and a mind that I simply didn't recognise. When I arrived at HQ, I would sit in my car, terrified at the prospect of starting the day. It would take a good fifteen minutes to get myself together.

I forced myself to carry on, never once taking a day off work. I'm sure people could tell that I'd been crying, even though I would use special eye-drops to try and hide it and reapply my make-up after tearful episodes. I had some very dark thoughts and it all felt so debilitating. Something clearly had to change.

At 51, I went to see my GP again, armed this time with a list of my symptoms. (I would highly recommend that people do this.) One of my friends had told me how life-changing HRT had been for her, and I wanted to try it. Within two weeks of starting treatment, I felt totally different. The panic and anxiety were both hugely reduced, and the tearfulness had stopped. One night I was sitting on the sofa with my family, and my son said, "Wow, Mum! You haven't shouted at Dad once!" It was a lovely moment and made me realise that I'd started to become my old self again.

I keep a close eye on how I feel. Sometimes my HRT prescription needs a little adjustment, and I still have the odd "Menopause Day", but "Mum's Magic Patches" (as my son very accurately calls them) basically do the trick.

I now work as an associate consultant, leading Menopause in the Workplace workshops and providing training for organisations to assist colleagues, line managers, HR, Occupational Health and leaders in understanding the menopause, so that they can help their female employees feel the best they can at work. I was even interviewed on the big red sofa on *BBC Breakfast*!

Of course, the menopause can affect all relationships – not only those at work. My top tips for getting through it? Share how you are feeling with your family and friends. Get support from your GP. See what treatment options work for you. You don't have to feel this way.

And remember, your symptoms won't last forever. I am living proof that things can be fabulous again – so try to enjoy your Second Spring!

Elsie Arkwright & Doris Rawbottom's story

(or *Hot Flushes and Red Cheeks*)

Me and Doris have been having problems,
Hot flushes and the like,
Experiencing terrible mood swings,
Waking up at night.

Tossing and turning all through night
And they like their sleep, do Bert and Len,
"It's time you got some sleeping pills,"
Bert said. "I were awake all night, again."

So me and Doris made an appointment,
I said, "Doctor won't mind if we share."
There we were, sat in waiting-room,
She said, "Have you seen who's over there,

"Smirking over her magazine?
That trollop from Number Four."
"I've decided to go back on pill," she said,
"What have you two come here for?"

"Ignore her," I said. "Pill indeed!
She's all of forty-five!"
"Well, she seems to do summat for our two,"
Said Doris. "With us two, they're barely alive."

Anyroad we went in to see doctor,
He were lovely with Doris and me,
He listened sympathetically,
Then sent us out with HRT.

Well, we got these patches from chemist,
Like see-through Elastoplast,
Stuck 'em on where it didn't show,
And a week later – what a contrast!

We were managing to get a good night's rest,
No need for hot milk and whisky,
Thank goodness they weren't doing what we'd feared,
We didn't want to feel frisky.

And Bert were sleeping like a top,
Doesn't get up before noon, no way,
I'm used to making bed round him
But got a shock when I threw back duvet.

He didn't move, he just snored on,
I were about to apprehend,
When I noticed that my HRT patch
Were stuck on his rear end.

I debated should I tell him,
Whether or not to say,
Then I thought, no, let him find out,
It won't be long before he goes out to play.

I'll tell you what, I had to smile,
He sneaked across to Number Four.
I thought, it won't be long before she finds out
Just what we went to doctor's for.

It weren't very long before he came home
Looking flustered, cheeks a bit red.
"I expect you'll be taking it off," I said,
"And sticking it back somewhere in bed.

"And if I were you, I'd start worrying,
Female hormones aren't good for men,
You might be neither use nor ornament
When you nip over road again."

Kate's story

I was 40 when I had my second child, with the tabloids nipping at my heels and warning me about the perils of older motherhood. Still recovering from a traumatic first birth twenty-two months earlier, this second one marked the start of an enormously stressful period of my life. Neither my partner nor I had relations nearby, nor did we have any friends with babies. We floundered, clinging desperately to the hope that our good-enough parenting was, indeed, good enough.

I know now that the quality of postnatal rest, especially with a birth in your forties, directly affects the quality of your perimenopause. Two births close together and an unsupported postnatal period did for my adrenals. Not that I noticed this for a while: I was too busy trying to get through the day without falling apart.

It's not easy being a carer to small children when starting the menopause; there is a very strong need to have time alone just at the point when you have to give yourself to others. And these little 'others' (bless them) make total bollocks of boundaries and energy reserves.

On returning to work, I developed a previously unknown desire to be seen. I wanted recognition; the invisibility of motherhood was eradicating my sense of self, so I went to look for it elsewhere. I ran a networking group for birth-workers, courses for therapists and my own Bodywork practice. I worked at my PR with a narcissism even I questioned, writing articles and blogs in any corner of time left over. How the hell did I manage all this? In retrospect, I'm surprised I didn't crack up much earlier.

Eventually, my poor, long-suffering adrenals blew the whistle. I was deeply fatigued, not sleeping more than a few hours a night and spending my days wandering and lost. Everything brought me inwards to focus on my inside world, sleeplessness and brain fog gently blanketing the outside world and rendering it fuzzy. Using Yoga Nidra was a godsend for exhaustion and restless legs, giving me an internal compass. I needed to listen to my body and my dreams.

During this time I was increasingly aware of the need to stop, and often talked about it, but actually doing it felt impossible. I remember seeing other women going on a Menopause Gap, and although I was in awe of their impressive self-care, I felt that if I stopped I would somehow cease to exist. Sjanie Hugo Wurlitzer, co-author (with Alexandra Pope) of *Wild Power*, says that her husband once said to her, "It takes a long time for a road train to stop between putting on the brakes and coming to a standstill." This remark gave me hope.

When I finally went to Alexandra Pope's menopause workshop in Malvern, I felt I had come home. This was my first experience of sitting in a circle with menopausal women and it is still my happiest place to be. Alexandra's beautiful teachings gave me the grounding from which I could understand myself and the hope that good things might lie ahead in the shape of a fresh Second Spring.

So there I was, busily letting go of my restrictive identities (as a professional, as a good-enough mum, as a 'nice' person) but I still hadn't really stopped. I still couldn't sleep, I worked in the evenings, skipped lunch and was awake at 4am with a fizzing alertness. My meditation practice, the yoga and the retreats were just more 'to-dos' on the list. The ultimate self-care of turning away from the world, which menopause asks us to do, was still beyond me. There's a big difference between knowing something and actually embodying it.

The turning point came following a Medicine Circle with Alexandra. She invited me to take a small dose of the rest my body so craved: fifteen minutes a day of doing nothing. Could I gift myself that? Incredibly, I wasn't sure I could. The earth would stop revolving, surely! Still, I put it in my diary, and the homeopathic dose began to work its magic. I had finally started to apply the brakes to the juggernaut.

My Bodywork practice was full, and my hands (my only tool) started to swell at the knuckles. I couldn't open the mayonnaise (and I like mayonnaise a lot). I don't really do regrets, but as a 19-year-old I didn't have much self-confidence and chose design instead of the fine art course which I really wanted to do. Since that time, my inner-critical voices had stopped me from exploring art for its own sake. The fact that my hands were losing their full range of movement showed me that I'd quite literally lost my grip on what gave me joy, and that if I continued to keep myself small by letting these inner-critics control me, it would eventually be too late, and I would never get to produce the art I longed to make. I heard the protest my knuckles were making loud and clear: "Don't put off your dreams for a future date. This is it. This is the only moment you have."

I had to let go of my work. I had to stop completely and allow the possibility of never going back. This was the moment of my surrender, allowing the identity that had nourished and sustained me for more than twenty-five years to be shrugged off and fall on the floor like an old coat.

Magic happened; no sooner had I conceived this desire than the finances came into place to ensure the bills were paid, and I knew that all would be well. Do you have to take time off from work/family to surrender in menopause? No. In a perfect world, should every woman be given the opportunity to do so if she wants to? Hell, yes!

Embarking on this six months of space was exquisitely sweet. Every task from washing-up to cleaning the loo gave me joy – because I was choosing to do it. I had a few rules:

- Only do pleasurable stuff. Reframe or delete if not.

- No thoughts of work/identity.

- Arrest your inner critic.

- Enjoy process.

- Abandon anything goal-orientated.

The only exception to this was the Medicine Circle training with Red School that lit up my heart. The timing fell so perfectly into my Menopause Gap, and I knew that this work was part of my future.

This period was a time of deep creativity. I learned to just 'be' with my family, allowing my own needs to be as important as theirs. In my free time, my inner world was inscribed firmly at the top of my list. I dropped into Biodynamic therapy again, and these weekly sessions became a well of nourishment. The Medicine Circles I received as part of my training soothed me each step of the way.

Returning from my Menopause Gap was, and still is, a tender process. I knew it would likely be a vulnerable time, and I took it slowly, trying to pace my emergence and resist both inner and outer demands to 'grow up' and 'get on with it'. I placed rigorous boundaries on my activities so that I didn't become overwhelmed again. Often I wore myself out, crashed and had to pull back, rest and recuperate.

What emerged was a sense of inner stillness. Arriving in Second Spring is a beautiful thing; I am myself, but without so much rubbish. I ask myself, "Does it connect me with love?" or on a less enlightened day, "Is it fun?" The rest can take a running jump.

I am deeply grateful to the menopause for the gifts it has delivered. After years of personal growth, I have finally learned to be kind to myself, to trust myself and to let go and love.

Jane H's story

Like many women my age, I had absolutely no idea what the menopause would entail beyond night sweats, hot flushes, being narky, and parts of my body shrivelling up. Such is the way it has been portrayed by urban myth and through the media. I started my periods when I was 14, and the only support I received from my mother was, "You know where the pads are." When my younger sister began hers at the age of 9, I was the one who had to explain everything. At least I had some knowledge from Biology classes, even though I didn't like what was happening to my body.

My own daughter has had the benefit of a supportive mother, attending an all-girls' school with emergency sanitary products on hand and going through a book on puberty with me. She was 11 when her periods started, and she was well prepared.

Until I started working in the area of menopause, I had no idea that there were 34 symptoms! On reflection, anxiety, depression and a growing lack of self-confidence came first for me. I wasn't myself and knew something was wrong – but didn't know what. I assumed that it was delayed grief: my husband had died when I was 41 and I started to feel different eight years later, when my daughter was 16. Having always been career-orientated, I lost interest in work, started having anxiety attacks whilst driving on the motorway, had narcoleptic episodes of fatigue during which I would just collapse without warning and burst into tears for no apparent reason. I recall picking my daughter up at the airport from a school trip: I'd been fine whilst she was away, but as soon as I saw her at Arrivals it was like a tear-tap had been turned on. Naturally, she was mortified.

On what would have been my 25th wedding anniversary, I remember walking around Manchester in a daze and bumping into a colleague who was visibly shocked at my appearance. Driving home, I started crying. Should I stop and try to recover, or continue home and retreat to my room? I chose the latter: I wasn't sure I'd be able to get back in the car and drive again otherwise.

A month later, I was on holiday and had time to think. Turning to the internet, I convinced myself that I was having a nervous breakdown and wrote a four-page document on how I was manifesting the key characteristics of one. Towards the end of the break, my then-boyfriend suggested meeting me and my daughter at the airport and taking us home. I said we would be fine. He arrived anyway – how sweet is that?! But I shoved him away, saying that we could manage by ourselves. All I wanted was to get back and retreat into myself. Talk about cutting off your nose to spite your face!

Back home, I couldn't get in: my key wasn't working. It was early on Sunday morning, and everything was closed, but I finally found the owner of an Open-All-Hours-We-Sell-Anything-And-Everything-Style shop pottering around in his pyjamas, and he sold me some WD40. It didn't work. I sent my daughter to a neighbour for our spare key…at which point I discovered that I was trying to get into the house with my office key!

I got myself an emergency appointment with the GP, handed over my four-page self-diagnosis and burst into tears. I was referred to The Priory to see a psychiatrist and have a twelve-week course of CBT. At no point did either the GP, the psychiatrist, various therapists or anyone at Occupational Health at work say, "We have a woman in her late forties here. Maybe she is menopausal." Nor did it cross my mind…until I started having night sweats and the penny finally dropped.

I had also totally gone off coffee, something which had happened when I was pregnant. Having been a vegetarian for over twenty-five years, I suddenly started craving baked salmon and black pudding. (I am from Bury so this craving wasn't as bizarre as it might appear.)

I discovered that my sleep consultant was going through similar dietary changes in her late forties/early fifties and had an inkling that hormones might be to blame. (During pregnancy I craved lasagne and cheese-and-onion pie in my first trimester, and honey-and-banana wholewheat butties in my third.)

The discomfort of my night sweats stopped me from functioning during the day – and this ended up being a catalyst for change in my life. I couldn't bear how much sweat I produced and struggled to get comfortable in bed. I thought, "There has to be a clothing solution to all this!" and also, "How on earth do women and their partners cope when sharing a bed?" Delirious through lack of sleep, and with no partner to talk to, I decided to jack in the day job (Senior Manager in Higher Education) and start a new career in fashion, with no prior experience other than making my own clothes at the weekend as a teenager, all set for a night of bopping. Like you do!

So I left my very well-paid and secure public-sector job, downsized to be mortgage-free, upset my daughter's lifestyle, sold a holiday home and self-funded a business in which I had no experience. Madness, yes, but that is the catchword of the menopause! What I do know is that I have solved my own problem of debilitating and uncomfortable night sweats, and solved it for other women, too. I call that a result, and a worthwhile endeavour.

Last November I discovered that I had vaginal atrophy, aka a dry vagina. I was having a Fleabag-style ongoing one-night-stand with a bloke who lives in Europe and is in a band. For a year and a half we hooked up whenever we were in the same country and vicinity. But one night, during foreplay, a pink, liquid discharge appeared. I no longer had periods, so something clearly wasn't right. I went straight to my wonderful GP, who gave me a pelvic examination and didn't seem unduly concerned. She said she suspected vaginal atrophy but would refer me anyway for an ultrasound. Best of all, she didn't judge my mid-life punk lifestyle.

The lady gynaecologist was a tad more judgemental – and somewhat uncommunicative. I had my scheduled smear at the same time as I had my investigative ultrasound, and although there were four female nurses/consultants in the room, another lady who was trained to do smears had to be drafted in. In the end there were five women looking on whilst my legs were in the air and my nether regions getting increasingly chilly.

I was prescribed an oestrogen-based vaginal cream – aka minor HRT – though no one told me what was being prescribed or why. My non-judgemental GP subsequently explained everything in detail and suggested that I supplement my weekly vaginal oestrogen insertion with a vaginal moisturiser. I have only very recently started to realise the importance of internal, as well as external, moisturisation.

Along the way, there have been some totally unexpected symptoms of the menopause: acne (not just on my face, but also on my back and my head); dry eyes; changes in diet; going completely bonkers without any warning; becoming a rare meat fanatic, having been a long-term vegetarian etc. etc.

My 21-year-old daughter keeps telling me that she now knows more about the menopause than anyone her age should. My take on this is that, like starting her periods, it's not going to come as a shock when her time comes, and she's lucky to have a mother who is so open and honest.

Nashi's story

I am a 50-year-old Albanian-British woman and am in reasonably good health.

I started to experience symptoms of the menopause when I was 36. The first thing I noticed was that my legs were cold during the night. It didn't matter how many covers I put on, or what the temperature was, I just couldn't get to sleep without wearing two pairs of socks. (My mother suffered from similar symptoms in her early fifties.) I had tests, but they all came back normal.

My bladder was also very sensitive. I had to go to the toilet at least every hour, and sometimes as often as every fifteen minutes. It left me exhausted the next day. Checks were done to see if there was any infection, but nothing showed up. Interestingly, I experienced some relief from both these symptoms in the days leading up to my period – and during menstruation itself.

My moods were all over the place. There were days when the tiniest thing would irritate me, and I had the urge to break glass. The sound of it shattering made me feel good for a split second. It was my 'Happiness Tablet'. During this time I was holding down a full-time job and looking after my family. I started to get hot flushes, which made me feel sick and drained. I often felt angry with my partner.

Three years ago, my cycle stopped, but my sleeping got worse. I hardly recognised myself. I was angry, emotional and didn't care what I said in the office. I once went into work having had only two hours' sleep. I would experience hot flushes during interviews: they were so intense, it felt as if I was having a seizure. All this had an impact on my work productivity, and it wasn't long before I discovered that my performance was being monitored. This just exacerbated my symptoms and my anger. I went to see my GP and asked for his help. Everything I looked at seemed dark, grim and dirty. I couldn't function anymore. The doctor was helpful and signed me off for a month. He suggested HRT, which I was happy to try, but after three weeks there was no improvement in my mood. I went to the doctor's again and asked to be referred to either a psychologist or a psychiatrist. It was then that the GP admitted that I'd been prescribed the wrong medication (oestrogen only).

After six weeks I returned to work and asked to move jobs within the unit. I was told, "We don't have any other roles for you." They said my performance was not as it should be and that I was therefore disqualified from any promotion.

The HRT was helping, but only very slowly. I developed panic attacks and anxiety and struggled to build new work relationships. My memory and concentration were both affected, and my confidence was crushed. I felt helpless and alone and was scared to talk to anyone. I couldn't believe that in my late forties I wasn't valued for what I did.

The panic attacks and anxiety worsened, and my life became hell. I walked around the house at night. My bed felt like it had thorns in it. It was as if the world was sliding from under my feet.

A few months later, I reached rock bottom. I could no longer function, either mentally or physically. I met my unit head and told her I was not well. I asked one final time for a job move, but all she did was put my name on the redeployment list. She also suggested that I see a doctor.

Since then I have been on antidepressants as well as HRT. I have not returned to work. I have been diagnosed with depression and PTSD and have had CBT, which has helped a little, especially with my sleep. It has also brought to the surface the political persecution and domestic violence I suffered in the past. It's extraordinary how these dreadful memories have been buried for decades.

I am now waiting for my health to improve. I deal with things better and don't blame other people for my suffering. My concentration and memory have improved. I hope that sharing my story will help other women going through the menopause.

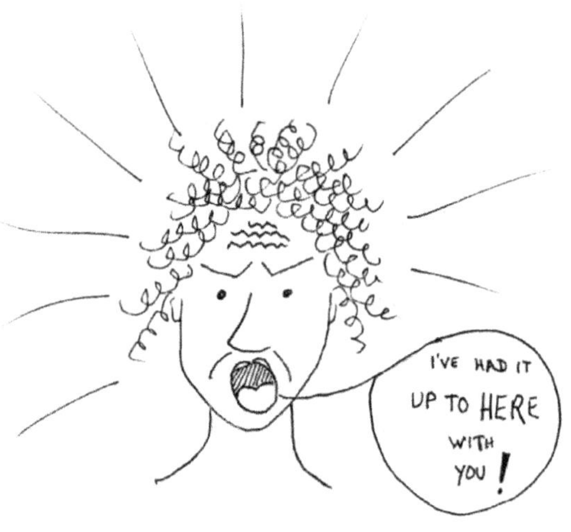

Jo's story

When you think of the menopause, you generally think of hot flushes. Most people aren't aware of all the other symptoms you can get: apparently there are more than thirty!

I've lived with mental illness in one form or another for most of my adult life. I saw my mum suffer from depression and panic attacks when she hit the menopause, although we didn't link the two at the time. I was unprepared when menopausal anxiety hit me.

I first became aware that these hormonal changes could affect mental health when I had a big meltdown at the age of 45. I had been struggling to ward off depression for several months. As is usually the case with depressives, I was trying to hide it from my loved ones, as I didn't want to "be a burden".

I had confided a little in my two best friends but hadn't told them the extent to which I was feeling fragile. Both told me to go and see the doctor, but I was sure I could beat it without medication, just like I'd done before.

I was at a music festival when it broke me. I normally feel quite safe in this situation, surrounded by good friends and the music that I love, but this time I couldn't handle it at all. I couldn't cope with having a conversation. I couldn't cope with watching the bands that normally sent me into my own little happy world. I couldn't cope with standing at the back of the room on my own, where I'd gone for a bit of breathing space. I had to escape.

I feigned a headache and said I was off to have a lie-down. I went to our hotel and cried and cried, admitting defeat to myself. Of course, there was no way I could hide it from anyone now.

My husband and friends were totally supportive, and I went to see my GP the following week. I assumed I would have to go back on antidepressants, something I hadn't needed to do for years. But my GP surprised me by saying that he thought the depression was menopause-related and asked how I felt about trying HRT instead. I was in such a bad place that I was prepared to give anything a go. I was actually quite relieved that I didn't have to take the antidepressants again.

But then a couple of years later I found that I was getting very anxious about things I couldn't control. I was aware that I was worrying too much but just couldn't stop the thoughts. I could see that my family found it difficult to understand when I was being irrational. It was so hard to cope with. I felt that my mind was totally out-of-control and that I was going a bit mad.

Then we had the year from hell: family illness, death and a road traffic accident. With all that – and more – going on, I figured that my anxiety could be explained, that it was justified.

My husband and I were forced to take some time out from our normally busy social calendar. We both needed some peace and quiet. We found more solitary pastimes in walking and reading and just being together.

When I felt ready to rejoin society, I found that my anxiety had mutated. I now had social anxiety! This was not like a panic attack, where you don't know what you're frightened of. I knew exactly what I was frightened of. I was scared that as I hadn't been out for so long, I would have nothing in common with my friends anymore – that I would have nothing to say and people would find me dull. I had also put on weight due to the menopause, so I didn't feel comfortable either in my body or my mind, which didn't help.

I wrote some articles on mental health and menopause on my blog, *Tea and Cake for the Soul*, and other women began to open up to me. It seemed we were all going through the same thing. Hearing one lady talk was like hearing an echo of what my own mind was saying. We both felt socially inept. But here we were having a meaningful conversation that helped us both so much. We were able to laugh (and cry) as we shared experiences and thoughts. We weren't socially inept at all; we had just changed.

So now I do go out – maybe not as often as before, but I enjoy myself and talk to my friends and nobody has ever walked out on a conversation with me yet. Maybe I'm not so dull after all! We are all batty old birds together!

I've focused here on the mental-health side of things, but I also suffered from hot flushes, which seemed to be more like a permanent (and very uncomfortable) increase in temperature. Long gone were the PJs, socks and hot water bottles at night. I slept naked and would wake up often, pulling the covers on and off throughout the night. Broken sleep left me irritable, which exacerbated my mental-health problems.

I remember my GP asking me which symptom I was most bothered by, and I said that I felt they were all connected. It was a vicious circle. I started on 1mg of HRT, which a couple of years later was increased to 2mg, and although I'm still far warmer than I was before the menopause, that has kept my heat to an acceptable level. My family begs me to put the heating on, but I see no need!

In the early days, I also had dry eyes and itchy skin. It felt like something was crawling over and under my skin. Thankfully that improved with the HRT.

Another horrible symptom I still suffer from is achy joints, particularly in my hands, something I always associated with much older people. I now focus on doing lots of joint-loosening exercises, such as qi gong, tai chi and yoga.

I find much of the menopause very frustrating but have made sure that I talk and write about it as much as possible to help other women know they're not alone. I think the more we can educate each other and tackle the subject with compassion and humour, the easier it becomes.

Joyce's story

The menopause – I have so much to say on the subject. I am an educator and professor in women's health and am very aware that women are not taught about it, so how are they supposed to deal with it when they don't know what might happen? The general perception of the menopause is that it is going to be horrendous. We need education and a positive view of it, especially postmenopause.

My own menopause was quite uneventful. When I was 42, I delivered twins after frozen embryo transfer, and after that had periods for a few years before things started to change. So my menopause symptoms got mixed up with all the stuff that happens when you are looking after three small children. For example, loss of libido. I'm not sure if this was down to the kids or the menopause. Tiredness – the same. But I did have some obvious menopausal symptoms, such as hot flushes and a change in my periods.

I have always been a very hot person, so being a bit hotter was bearable. I made sure I kept cool as much as I could. At the time, one of my students was doing a project on the menopause, and her conclusion was that exercise reduces hot flushes. I have always been an exercise addict, but having kids made finding the time for it harder, so I used the menopause as an excuse to get back into it. I am now an ambassador for *This Girl Can*, the UK campaign to encourage women to exercise. I started running in my late forties and love it to this day. I am very slow but relish the feeling it gives me of clearing my brain. Talking of which, that's how I describe myself postmenopause: I have a clear brain. It really is as if a cloud has been lifted. Until the menopause, I never realised how up and down I felt each month as I went through my menstrual cycle. I think for half of each month I was too emotional and maybe a bit mad. Postmenopause I even contacted two ex-boyfriends and apologised for being so crazy when I was younger…

I did have some vaginal dryness and itching, and this was treated with oestrogen pessaries. I only had to use them for about a year and then things got back to normal.

Probably the worst thing for me was the change in my periods. They had always been quite light and short, but for the two years before they finally stopped, they were all over the place and incredibly painful. I had several heavy bleeds lasting over two weeks. I know for some women this problem can continue for a long time.

I totally appreciate that every woman is different: through puberty, through our menstrual cycles and through the menopause. But I strongly believe that after menopause we need to regain control of our lives. We spend so much time looking after everyone else, and the menopause is a really good time to reset. If we have let things slip, we have to get back on track with our nutrition, exercise, sleep and mental health. If these four pillars of wellbeing are in order and we are still getting menopausal symptoms, we should seek medical help. However, the quality of GPs varies, so it might take time to find a sympathetic doctor. Don't suffer in silence.

My mission is to educate women about the menopause. Many google their symptoms, but only after they have started suffering. Some don't realise that their symptoms are due to the menopause, such as depression. We need women to be armed with menopause knowledge before symptoms start. And the menopause can begin in our late thirties or early forties.

Postmenopause gives us freedom from our reproductive ties. No more periods, no more premenstrual syndrome, no more contraception. For me, my fifties have been the most productive years of my life. My mind seems sharper than it's ever been. I am so full of ideas. I am more level. And I am calmer.

Bring on the menopause: let's celebrate this wonderful stage in our lives!

Lesley-ann's story

When I was a little girl, my dad used to say that he could see Christmas lights in my eyes. When I was sad, my lights dimmed, and my dad always knew. Lately I have lost those lights. Damn the menopause!

I was toddling along fine, experimenting with a variety of different HRT combinations – and then The Great HRT Shortage of 2019 hit. My GP told me, "I'm sorry, but there are no suitable HRT drugs in stock." I headed home in disbelief to contemplate an HRT-free existence. How would I juggle flushes, migraines, low mood, menopausal fog, teenagers, a husband and work?

There appeared to be no information or support on how to cope with HRT Cold Turkey. I came up with the solution of gritting my teeth and exercising. Plan B was always available, which was to sit down in a heap and cry!

I am usually a glass-half-full person, but I have found all this very difficult – constantly being hit by feelings of overwhelm and anxiety. Home was the easy part. I'd hoped I'd stored up some wife/mum points after years of devotion, and my family have shown me love and kindness in the main. I think that's quite a win, given that I spend most of my time living in a chaotic boys' world. Work has been much more of a challenge. I'm in mental health and often feel completely out-of-my-depth as I struggle with my own turbulent emotions. I spoke to my manager about it, but he's a young man, and it was obvious that discussing my menopause with him was a case of oversharing! He reminded me that I was older than his mum! We discussed how I couldn't realistically take on extra responsibilities, due to the anxiety this would cause me. He took this on board, but I felt that I was a disappointment, both to myself and him.

The flushes mean that I often have sweaty hair, and buying a new work-wardrobe full of natural fabrics has meant that I am now "that woman with a crumpled linen dress and a red head". Learning new stuff has been a nightmare: I struggle to remember what I did yesterday!

I have never been much of a crier, but now feel close to tears most days, especially when I feel overwhelmed.

And so I carry on along the bumpy road of menopause. I feel that the need for kindness in my life has never been greater! I miss 'me' – the person I was. I miss my Christmas lights...

Karen T's story

I was in my mid-forties when I first realised that I might be perimenopausal. I was watching TV and suddenly became aware of feeling very hot. For some years I had joked about looking forward to the menopause, because for most of my life I have had cold hands and feet, and I felt it would be nice to be warm for a change.

Of course, it's not like that at all. That first flush was a deeply unwelcome sensation of suffocating heat, and I had to go and stand outside in the cool evening air just to prove to myself that I could still breathe. Subsequent hot flushes were (and still are) equally unpleasant: they started with a brief sensation of nausea, then a tingling, fizzing feeling somewhere in my solar plexus, followed by an explosion of sudden heat that released a sometimes-drenching amount of sweat.

During my thirties, I had never had a day's trouble with periods: they were reasonably regular and easy to manage. I actually enjoyed the predictability of my cycle. As a textile artist, I liked working with the different energies it afforded: at mid-cycle, when I was ovulating, I was more energetic and outward-looking and could easily come up with new ideas and designs. At the end of the cycle, when I was menstruating, I had less physical energy but felt more reflective and meditative and could uncover more layers of meaning in my work. I felt that working in harmony with my body and the different energies of its cyclical rhythms enriched my life.

The first time I missed a period, aged about 44, I bought a pregnancy test, and took it with a mixture of dread and excitement. I had never wanted children, but there was a point in my early forties when I realised that if I was ever going to be anyone's mother, it was probably now or never. At that time, I was having recurring dreams about eggs, which I now realise came directly from my failing ovaries: I dreamed I bought a box of eggs from the supermarket, but when I got it home, the eggs were either missing, broken, bad or hard-boiled. When the pregnancy test was negative, I wondered whether this was the shape of things to come. I had read that periods can become 'slightly irregular' as a woman nears the menopause. What an understatement that turned out to be!

Over the next few years, I had every kind of horrendous period imaginable: too long (some lasted three or four weeks); too short (less than a day); too heavy (I had never seen so much blood); too light (might as well not have happened); too frequent (every two weeks); too infrequent (every three or four months); and too painful (I once fainted from the intensity of period pain). I visited the doctor only once during this time, when it was discovered that my iron levels had become seriously low. I resisted HRT because I assumed that it would just delay the inevitable transition and I didn't ever want to go through this again. The doctor didn't really explain to me how HRT worked, or how it might help. She shrugged and said we all had to go through the menopause at some point.

Like most other working-class women, I continued to suffer in silence. I had dry skin, a burning mouth, dry eyes, crashing fatigue, difficulty sleeping and concentrating, brain fog, dizziness, headaches, muscle cramps and anxiety. My usual deodorant was ineffective, and I noticed that I was sweating more profusely and that the sweat smelt more acidic. In fact, my whole body smelt different. My skin had suddenly become dry and seemed much looser than before. Most troubling of all was the loss of my energy cycle. I was no longer experiencing the highs of ovulation and the lows of menstruation, but was caught somewhere in-between in a shadowy limbo that was neither one thing nor the other. I hardly knew myself anymore.

The one thing that did seriously alarm me was the rage I felt. For a time, I was consumed by a boiling, white-hot, incandescent anger that was completely unfamiliar and out-of-character. I could cheerfully have killed any man who came within a few feet of me. I hated everyone and could barely think straight. I felt as if I needed to stand on a high mountain and rail at the sky until my voice gave up.

I've since heard that this is quite common, but I was totally unprepared for it. I have no sisters, and my mother had undergone a hysterectomy at the age of 44, so I felt alone and bewildered as I wrestled with the whole range of weird things my mind and body were suddenly doing.

I read somewhere that a girl's brain is rewired at puberty, and that the cycling hormones programme her to nurture others in preparation for motherhood. This is particularly cruel when it happens to girls who know they don't want, or will never have, children. When the cycle of oestrogen and progesterone ends at menopause, the brain is wired back to the way it was before puberty. At that point we feel as if we have suddenly woken up to the fact that we've given other people (often men) the best years of our life.

Little wonder, once the rage had passed, that I became uncharacteristically weepy. It felt as if I were grieving for everything that I thought I had lost, including my reliable cycle, my emotional equilibrium, my attractiveness and my youth. I wished, more than anything, that I could have talked to someone about what was happening to me. Even other women my age seemed reluctant to discuss it. Why are we encouraged to be so silent about what happens to our bodies?

One of the many things that we remain silent about is how long this goes on for. Ten years later, I'm discomfited to find that I'm still having disruptive symptoms: hot flushes and night sweats; burning mouth and fatigue; headaches; difficulty concentrating; trouble sleeping. The one benefit I can see is that my periods, so problematic towards the end, finally stopped altogether a couple of years ago, and my emotional equilibrium is now beginning to settle. I'm starting to enjoy not having to carry emergency sanitary protection wherever I go, and there's no longer any danger of a period arriving on, say, the first day of a holiday.

I actually feel that I've got through the menopause quite lightly. Most of it was inconvenient and bewildering, rather than an illness needing to be medicated. That limbo-like position – where I felt neither the surge of ovulation nor the doldrums of menstruation – has morphed into a stability, similar to the end-of-cycle introspection which I used to experience, but without the inconvenience and pain of bleeding. That quiet, contemplative state has become more or less permanent, and I am learning to accept it.

The amazing thing about women is that they can bear so much physical and emotional discomfort while remaining relatively sane and stoical. I am at last approaching a place where I can say I am nearly OK, which is often as good as it gets.

Isabel's story

Am I menopausal? I honestly don't know, because my periods are still chemically regulated. And I have no road-map: my mum had a hysterectomy for medical reasons well before the menopause, and we never really talked about what it meant for her. But am I perimenopausal? Let me count the ways…

- Inexplicable inability to think of a word or a name when I need it? Tick. Very inconvenient at work, that one. Kids also mystified why I can't remember the names for simple things.

- Night sweats? Tick. Not yet full flushes during the day, though. I would quite happily skip those.

- Sudden bouts of exhaustion? Tick. Sometimes I can't get my own body up the stairs.

- Waves of hormones leading to sudden wish to weep or explode? Tick.

- Sudden arrival of extra weight? Tick. By the way, if my metabolism has slowed down, why do I still get hungry?

- Facial outbreaks? Tick. Also the onset of rosacea, which is sporadic, but not fun, and just makes my kids ask why I've got a red face. Last year I got what appeared to be the sort of sunburn that comes from failing to apply sunblock. I felt like an idiot: I was slathered in factor 50. Now at least I know why.

- I'm also going to attribute my regular need for chocolate – preferably plain chocolate – to being perimenopausal. It's just part of the hormonal management, right?

Luckily all this is hitting when I don't really give a monkey's what people think. If I can't find the right word, then so what? But there's no getting away from that moment in a meeting (and my meetings are often round a table full of men) when the next word (or the entire rest of the sentence) completely disappears. Just when I want the right word for exactly the right impact, I find ten faces looking at me expectantly. My inner monologue goes something like this: "Oh look! All those words have floated away. I have no idea what I was going to say. Look at all those people staring at me, waiting for the next word. Hmm, better come up with a word. Doesn't matter whether it's the right one. Just say something and you'll at least finish your sentence." Thanks to my awareness of menopausal symptoms, I don't have to suffer an inner monologue that says, "You idiot! You're losing your mind!" That said, I could do with it not occurring too frequently. I'm lucky to have one female colleague a couple of years older than I am, who regularly can't find the right word, and it's just an unspoken agreement that we gloss over it. We both know why it happens: it doesn't require comment.

The exhaustion and hormonal rages are more of a challenge, but OK if I can save the worst of the effects till home-time. Lots of deep breaths are required when I'm irrationally furious with the kids, but I hope I don't progress to sudden weeping fits in the workplace...

At this stage, then, my symptoms are more inconvenient than utterly debilitating. I'll be keeping my antennae tuned in for more, and for tips from others on how to manage them.

The irony of all this is that while I am preparing for the menopause, one of my kids is preparing for puberty. There are some interesting parallels. We are both dealing with skin issues, weepiness and swamps of hormones. I'm pleased to report that we talk a lot, so we'll be educating one another. I will certainly be talking to her a lot more than my mum talked to me…

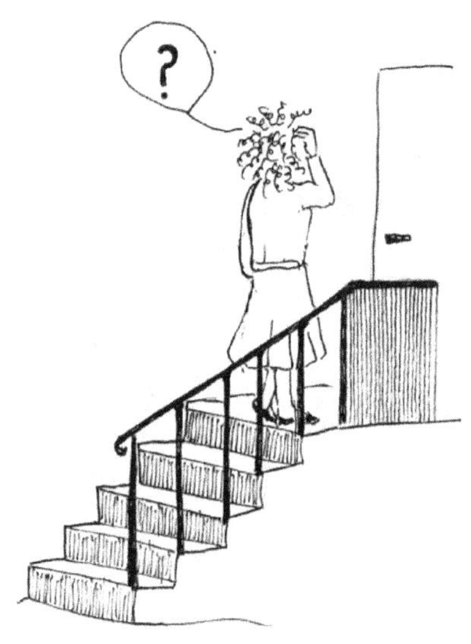

Karen K's story

I can pinpoint, almost to the day, when my menopause story started. It was December 2003, and after bleeding continuously since giving birth to my son nine months earlier, I had a hysterectomy at the age of 34. I retained my ovaries and was sent on my way after the operation with the advice that I would go into menopause "at the normal time". I didn't know when "the normal time" was and to be honest, it didn't occur to me to ask. It was a long way off, and nothing for me to worry about.

However, despite my hysterectomy, my periods continued. This frightened me: my mind was filled with all sorts of terrifying cancer-related scenarios, and as a young mum with two small children, my fear about what was going on was enormous. I went to my GP, who told me not to be "ridiculous". "You can't be having periods," he said. "You've had your womb removed." His reaction was upsetting and unhelpful and I left feeling scared and confused, with no idea what was wrong. I looked elsewhere for help. I trawled the internet for information on bleeding post-hysterectomy. The most relevant search led me to email the British Menopause Society, but what was happening to me baffled them, too.

We moved to Germany, and I found a gynaecologist who was able to work out what was wrong. My previous caesarean section had left some of my cervix scarred onto the side of my bladder and rather than risk any long-term complications by removing this, my hysterectomy surgeon had left it behind. I was unaware that any of this had happened but finally I was able to have keyhole surgery to solve the problem.

Throughout all this, I had begun to experience symptoms which I now recognise as menopause-related. They had started just a couple of weeks after the operation, but I didn't pick up on them immediately because I was more concerned about the unexpected bleeding.

I suffered from hot flushes so severe that I would be left embarrassingly drenched. Then there were the low moods, and insomnia so debilitating that I struggled by on only two or three hours' sleep each night. Add to that fatigue, sore joints, heart palpitations, headaches, dizziness and brain fog. I didn't know what was happening to me and, rather more worryingly, neither did the doctors.

There was always an explanation for each symptom, but never a look at the symptoms as a package. The sweats were apparently because we'd been living in Riyadh at the time, even when I argued that I kept the air-conditioning set to Glasgow temperatures! When the flushes continued in Germany, I was treated for hyperhidrosis (excessive sweating) and everything dried up except the flushes! My insomnia, I was told, was because I had two small children, and nobody gets much sleep then. (It continued until last year.) I was informed that I was suffering an anxious reaction to continuing to have periods following my hysterectomy, but even after that was resolved, the symptoms remained.

No matter which symptom I went with, I was given a seemingly reasonable explanation as to why I was suffering from it. Back then, I didn't know enough (anything!) about the menopause to enable me to recognise what was happening and argue my case.

There were countless trips to see the doctor, and I dreaded every single one of them. Eventually, nine years after the hysterectomy, a GP suggested that I might be experiencing menopausal symptoms. However, blood tests failed to support this theory. I now know that these tests can be unreliable because of fluctuating hormone levels. We discussed HRT as an option, but this was dismissed because I suffer from migraines.

My lack of knowledge, together with my assumption that GPs know more than their patients, stopped me from taking this any further and I decided to look for other ways to deal with my symptoms.

Spending more money than we could afford, I tried all sorts of things to get relief, with some remedies proving more successful than others. There are lots of products on the market targeted at menopausal women and, in my desperation, I tried many of them. This route is expensive though, and not sustainable long-term, so I began to look for answers once again. I found one of many Facebook groups where menopausal women could ask questions and get support. It was so refreshing – women talking about the menopause! I no longer felt quite so alone.

As I became more involved in the group, I was asked to moderate the company's new community forum, set up specifically to help women cope with symptoms of the menopause. I had access to experts on the site and could ask them all sorts of questions.

I soon discovered that HRT actually was an option for me, if I took it via transdermal patches or gel. I also had a new GP, and armed with my new information I asked him about getting HRT patches. He was sympathetic and informed, and he listened. Best of all, he agreed. We talked about the possible side effects of HRT, including bloating, breast tenderness and an increase in headaches, but he also explained the benefits: future-proofing my bones against osteoporosis and helping to protect my heart from coronary heart disease. I felt I had finally found a doctor who knew about the menopause.

Nine months on from my first prescription, I am a different woman. My life has been transformed. In fact, I now feel so good that it hardly seems possible that I endured nearly sixteen years of symptoms. My husband is delighted (and relieved) to see the difference in me, and my teenage boys are thrilled to have a calmer and much less shouty mother.

Every woman has her own menopause story to tell. None of what I've described is a bid for sympathy – it's simply what happened to me, and I'm sharing it in the hope that it may help other women. It's also why I'm one of the co-founders of Pausitivity, a menopause campaign started in July 2019 to provide women with information about menopause symptoms on a poster: a simple concept to prompt them to ask questions and enable them to have discussions about all things menopausal with the people in their lives. Knowing our campaign is already having this effect is very powerful. GPs, politicians, organisations, women, men – people from all walks of life are joining in to make menopause something we can talk about at last.

I believe that if I had known the symptoms, if I had known that despite keeping my ovaries during my hysterectomy I was likely to experience an early menopause, if I had known more about the HRT treatments available, I would have been better placed to identify what was happening to me and I'd have had the knowledge I needed to raise my concerns. I wouldn't have suffered for so long.

Thanks to the changes that are finally beginning to happen, we are talking about menopause and helping others to have the conversations that I found so difficult. I have high hopes that future generations of women will be far better informed and much more able to choose the way they direct their own menopause stories.

Fianna's story

The menopause crept up on me through the back door. I'm not exactly sure when it started, but it has changed both my mind and my body.

Hot flushes and my widening waist made me unsure, tentative and anxious. Brain fog was probably the worst symptom, affecting my work and making me feel out-of-control.

One day at work, I listened to my colleagues talking about 'The Change'. The moaning and groaning was deafening. I decided I could either join in and feel depressed or do something constructive to lessen the symptoms. I wasn't going down without a fight!

I was 50 and my children were now more independent, so I signed up to the gym and used a personal trainer. Slowly but surely, I started to regain my lost confidence and, encouraged by my trainer, began believing in myself and getting back into shape.

I was realistic. I knew I would never have the body of an 18-year-old again, but I felt I could certainly tone up and lose a stone or so. And I have. The feeling I get from swimming, walking, and doing cardio and weights has helped me battle my insecurities and focus on something positive. The 'high' I feel after exercise is great. I eat healthily but allow myself the odd treat, and my various menopausal symptoms have lessened. I have more confidence after losing my excess weight and no longer care what others think of me. I am also taking some supplements prescribed by a nutritionist, which is helping to balance my moods.

My husband works away, I am a busy working mum, and I still struggle with various symptoms from time to time. But I have learned to take a step back: to STOP and BREATHE. Half the battle is to allow myself some space to work through the symptoms I'm experiencing and slow down, because I just can't multitask like I used to.

The menopause has most definitely changed me, and sometimes I miss my former self. But there is no going back…

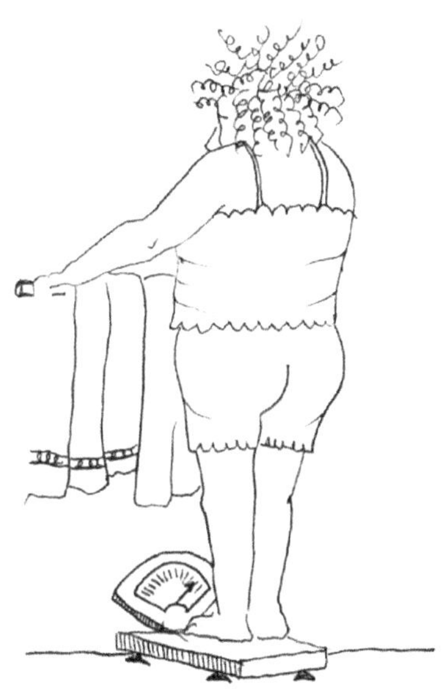

Lucy's story

My experience of menopause was like nothing I'd ever heard of. Like a hormonal tornado, it blew me off my feet, turned my life upside-down and landed me in a new city with a new partner and a radically different lifestyle.

What happened? A huge surge in sex drive, the likes of which I'd never before experienced but which whirled into my life and totally took over. While I was going through it – the peak lasted about eight months – friends would joke at the unfairness of their migraines compared with my wild sex life, but I warned them to be careful what they wished for. When a force that strong takes over your life, it leaves little time for anything else. I was like a stereotypical teenage boy, unable to focus on anything except my next fix and, for the first time, I understood why sex is at the base of Maslow's hierarchy.

I'd always had a healthy sex drive but like most people it had taken a dip after I had children, and my husband and I had slipped into the familiar once-a-week-to-keep-things-ticking-over routine.

We lived in a pretty riverside town where I home-schooled our children. We'd moved there to balance my desire to be out of London with my husband's commute to the city, and I had little in common with the people who lived near us, but kept myself stimulated writing a couple of blogs which allowed me to connect with kindred spirits around the world while I educated our kids.

My husband had a highly-paid job that didn't make him happy, but I'd long since given up trying to persuade him to find something that made him less miserable. I foresaw a comfortable life together after the children left home, with me going back to my therapy work and the two of us taking nice holidays a few times a year.

My periods had become less regular during my late thirties and into my forties, and I was grateful that the pre-menstrual mood symptoms I'd experienced in my younger years had mostly stopped by my mid-thirties. I thought little about either my hormones or my periods, which would arrive between a few weeks and several months apart, and I anticipated them gradually and uneventfully phasing out.

In the months preceding my 47th birthday, I started to spend more time listening to rock music with my 14-year-old daughter and found myself reminiscing about my teen and twenty-something years. I felt happy that my daughter had so much excitement ahead of her but also a little sad that the most fun and passionate times of my life were behind me.

Then, a month before I turned 47, I went on a weekend away with a girlfriend. We found ourselves dancing in a bar filled with friendly thirty-something men and I suddenly realised that not only was I extremely attracted to some of them, but that the attraction was reciprocated.

Looking back, this feeling of being aware of (mostly younger) men around me had been building over the preceding months, but it wasn't until my break away with my friend that I realised what was happening. Suddenly I began noticing men absolutely everywhere and found myself obsessed with wanting to kiss them (and more).

A week later, I was sitting in the cinema with my husband and 12-year-old son when I had a startling epiphany. I realised that I no longer wanted to be married. My mother had divorced three times and it'd always been a point of pride for me that, unlike her, I would make a success of my marriage. I'd given up paid work to home-educate our children and had never imagined a future without my husband, financial or otherwise. And now, suddenly, it was as if I was standing in the middle of a glass cake-stand, and someone had taken the lid off. I reeled in shock as I took in a new reality – a faraway, unknown wilderness beyond walls which I hadn't even known were imprisoning me.

When I got home from the cinema, I did what I always do when I feel off-balance – I meditated. As I did so, my inner wisdom quietly told me not to take hasty action, but to meditate regularly and not to share my thoughts with anyone until I was clearer about what I wanted.

There followed a summer in which I could barely function for thinking about sex. Everywhere I went, I imagined what it would be like to be in bed surrounded by men. On the motorway I would imagine stopping at service stations with van drivers. Popping to the corner shop I'd have to avoid eye contact with local dads. At the gym I'd have to use a cross-trainer next to the window to avoid drooling over the toned hunks working out beside me. And I went to the gym a lot. I discovered that a hard workout was just about the only way to achieve temporary respite from my raging hormones.

I mentioned what was going on to a few close friends, and one admitted to lusting after men for a while in the run-up to her divorce, but no one seemed to have experienced anything on the scale that was happening to me. In my desperation, I reached for google, where to my intense relief I finally found some answers.

Joanna Meriwether, a coach in the US, described my experience exactly. I won't try and share her story here, as she does a wonderful job of it on her website. (See *Helpful*

Resources and Contacts page at the back of this book.) Joanna was my saviour. Reading her story and the testimonials of other women she had worked with made me feel, if not sane again, then at least a whole lot less crazy.

She explained that for women like us, the perimenopause is characterised by an intense spike in libido, probably as our bodies go on one last, all-out drive to get pregnant. Although not a scientist, Joanna also suspects that we give off pheromones that make us attractive to men, including much younger men. This certainly reflected my own experience.

Via a series of remote coaching sessions, Joanna lovingly helped me find direction in my life. I did end up leaving my husband, which was obviously painful for us both, but thankfully we were able to handle the divorce process without bitterness and we remain good friends and co-parents to our teenage children.

I moved to a vibrant city on the coast where I feel totally at home and surrounded by my tribe – a stark contrast to the champagne suburb I left. My husband moved back to London and – although he's never been the optimist I am – I like to think that we're both happier now.

I had my last period four months before my 48th birthday. That was eighteen months ago, and I'm happy to say I haven't experienced any other menopausal symptoms, although I keep plenty of lube to hand, in case the dryness my older friends warn of should ever strike!

My libido has gradually returned to a manageable level, so I'm now able to maintain a very satisfying relationship with my (equally satisfied!) boyfriend.

I was delighted to come across the first volume of *The Menopause Monologues* – I think it's really important that women talk about their experiences so that they can better support one another. And when I realised that no one had shared a story like mine, I was keen to contribute to this second book, because although what happened to me might be rare, I'm not the only one, and when your libido suddenly takes over your life, you need all the support you can get!

Totes' story

Hi, my name is Totes and I'm perimenopausal. It sounds like the opening line from an Alcoholics Anonymous meeting, doesn't it? I'm 47 but my blog bio would inform you that I'm 43. This is an oversight but one that I keep neglecting to rectify.

Menopause or perimenopause – call it what you will – is a bit rubbish, but what can you do about it? You can share all those disturbing memes on social media about the Seven Dwarves of the Menopause and the Menopause Fairy, which portray women as dried-up and itchy has-beens, or you can find more productive ways of making yourself feel better. Personally, I can't stand the 'laughter is the best medicine' attitude, because frankly the symptoms of the menopause aren't very funny. How does it help our cause when women are portrayed like Cissie & Ada from the seventies' TV programme? Menopause seems to be one of the last bastions in which mocking the afflicted is actively encouraged.

In my early forties, when my children were still very small, I had really bad mood swings. I put them down to PMT and went to see my doctor. I'd had three pregnancies close together and before this had spent over fifteen years having injections for birth control. Because of this, I hadn't had any periods in a very long time, so I thought I'd simply forgotten what it felt like to have normal hormonal fluctuations. To illustrate my point, I told the doctor that my husband called me his "little pit viper" or "Rottweiler".

I was prescribed antidepressants, which I happily tried because I didn't want to be angry all the time, but with hindsight, I don't think that they were the answer. I was probably just experiencing a drop in my oestrogen levels and was angry at my husband because he's often a bit of an idiot. (Later, when I set up a Facebook group aimed at menopausal women, I discovered that antidepressants seemed to be handed out to them like sweets.)

Anyway, I loathed the antidepressants, which made me feel numb and dead behind the eyes, so against my doctor's advice I weaned myself off them. For the last two years, I've also had joint pain (particularly hip pain) and then the final nail in the coffin was the brain fog. I actually began to question whether I had dementia. I could barely string a sentence together because I couldn't recall simple words. Even when writing, I'd have a complete block and would have to look things up. I've also been diagnosed with a vitamin B12 deficiency, and often struggle to know which symptom I should attribute to which condition, given that they share so many.

I was much more compliant when I was younger – eager to please and needing to be liked – but have recently become far less tolerant. That sounds like a negative, but actually it has its virtues. About four years ago, I started writing a blog about my life as a woman of a certain age. Amongst other things, it covers what it's really like to parent three young children, and it has been a real outlet for me. I can't bear the social media lies about the perfect family and wanted to bring a bit more honesty and humour to the genre of the parenting blog.

Because I find it difficult to write about only one topic, I also tackle other subjects, such as politics and fashion. I photograph what I'm wearing most days (which, as time has gone by, has become more and more outlandish) and refuse to blend into the background and age gracefully. I want to be more than just someone's wife and mother, wearing something tasteful, expensive and drab. I don't have a proper job anymore because I'm pretty much unemployable, so I'm trying to write a dark but humorous novel about a perimenopausal blogger. The menopause seems to rob you of your confidence, so stepping out of your comfort zone can be very hard, but I have tried to say yes to new things, even when I've not been particularly confident about doing so. This has led to some pretty unspectacular appearances on television and radio, and also to a very drunken attempt at public speaking.

I also run. A lot. Running keeps me sane. I began running just before I had my children and now I've upped my game and have just completed my tenth marathon. I'm by no means a natural athlete. I spent most of my twenties in clubs, smoking and taking recreational drugs. I did no exercise until I needed to lose weight in my mid-thirties. However, running has helped me cope with my anxiety, which is just one of the many wonderful symptoms of perimenopause. It also gave me another subject for my blog, which in turn led me to set up an online virtual community for runners of all abilities. It has just reached twenty-five thousand members and become UK Athletics affiliated.

I have recently started HRT and now take a plethora of supplements. I hardly recognise the person I was in my twenties and thirties. I'm still me – but different…

Clare S's story

It is a cold November morning, the snow on the hillside is glistening in the sunlight and I'm lying on a hospital bed wondering how on earth I ended up here. My two children and husband are by my side, and I hear my 9-year-old say, "Will you be alright, Mum?" And I think to myself, "I bloody well hope so, because the last seven years have been the pits!"

I'm 39 and just about to have a hysterectomy to remove my womb and ovaries. Seven years earlier, I'd given birth to my second daughter, and accepted that it would take time for the hormones to settle down and the fatigue to improve (especially given the sleepless nights). But a year later I was still not feeling 'right'. My moods were erratic, and I was starting to get unpleasant stomach pains. I was told that it was all fine: the post-baby hormones were apparently just taking a little longer than usual to settle, and the stomach pains were nothing to worry about.

The fatigue worsened over the coming years. Twice I missed picking the children up from school as I was fast asleep on the settee. I started to opt out of social events because I just wanted to be at home in bed. Blood tests didn't show any medical cause, but I became convinced I had ME or chronic fatigue syndrome.

Mood swings, together with frightening outbursts of anger and difficulties with both my concentration and memory, made me think I had a brain tumour. But I didn't. The doctors said so.

My periods became heavier and my cycle was as erratic as my moods. I resorted to carrying spare underwear and sanitary towels with me at all times. Tampons alone definitely weren't sufficient. My stomach pains were now more severe, and I was worried I had womb cancer. But I didn't. The doctors said so. They suggested I take the contraceptive pill to control the pain and stabilise my cycle.

On two occasions I flooded at work, staining the fabric seat. Have you ever tried explaining that one away to your colleagues? Or walked through a busy office with blood showing through your clothes? And still the stomach pain increased. The doctors booked me in for an ultrasound, but the results didn't show anything.

I noticed that my heart was beginning to race. Was it due to the mood swings, anger, brain fog, the feeling that I was losing control? My anxiety levels rocketed, and I had two panic attacks close together. The doctors suggested beta blockers.

By now I was frightened. I knew that there was something wrong with me. Gone was the level-headed, confident, sociable woman I'd once been. I no longer recognised myself – and neither did my husband. All this was taking a toll on our relationship, not helped by my lack of libido and the increasingly unbearable pain of intercourse.

But there was nothing wrong with me. The doctors said so. They offered me antidepressants.

I felt so alone.

Over a period of seven years, I saw seven doctors. My symptoms were constantly dismissed, and I resorted to excessive drinking and smoking to help dampen the fear and lessen the pain.

One day I poured my heart out to a friend a few years older than me, and she suggested that the symptoms could be due to menopause. Menopause? The word wasn't even in my vocabulary! I was in my thirties, for goodness sake! Encouraged by my husband, I went private and saw an endocrinologist, who quickly confirmed that I was well into perimenopause, and suggested that the pain could be due to endometriosis. Further tests indicated that this was indeed the case and that the adhesions were attached to my ovaries and bowel. No wonder I was in so much pain...

Armed with this information, I returned to my doctor, waving the results in front of his face. Because of my age, he had never considered that I could be menopausal! He'd seen me as a neurotic woman, increasingly unable to cope with her life.

Nonchalantly, he asked if I had private health insurance, as the NHS wouldn't give me a hysterectomy at my age. Luckily, I did – and very soon after that I was lying on that hospital bed with my family by my side, ready for surgery. I couldn't wait…

Following the operation, I was offered HRT. The pill didn't suit me, but I could tolerate patches and soon I was feeling a lot better. Much more like my old self. However, it was recommended that I shouldn't continue taking the HRT for more than ten years, so I vowed that once I reached the age of 50, I would wean myself off it very gently. I didn't want to go back to feeling the way I did before the hysterectomy. So when the time came, that's what I did. I changed my nutrition and lifestyle, and for a while all went well.

And then my world was turned upside-down. My eldest daughter was diagnosed with cancer, and eighteen months later she left us. Every single symptom attributed to the menopause returned. The anxiety was so great that I considered ending my life on more than one occasion.

Why didn't I go back on HRT, given that I knew it could help me? Because around this time the Women's Health Initiative report suggested it wouldn't be a good idea. I'd been taking HRT for twelve years, and the risks were considered high if I continued. I had to ride the storm yet again.

So, what changed? Well, I was walking my dog through the woods one day, and it occurred to me that she didn't worry about the past or the future: she simply lived in the now. Something I'd forgotten how to do. I also realised that I owed it to my other daughter to do just that. So I reapplied everything I'd learned in the past and took back control of my life. I refused to let the menopause define me.

I'll soon be 66. Those early menopause years were a long time ago, but the memory of them still lingers. My message to others would be to research the options available and make the right choices. Most importantly, know that there is a bright light waiting for you on the other side. Don't hanker after the person you used to be. Instead, look forward to the strong, confident woman you can become.

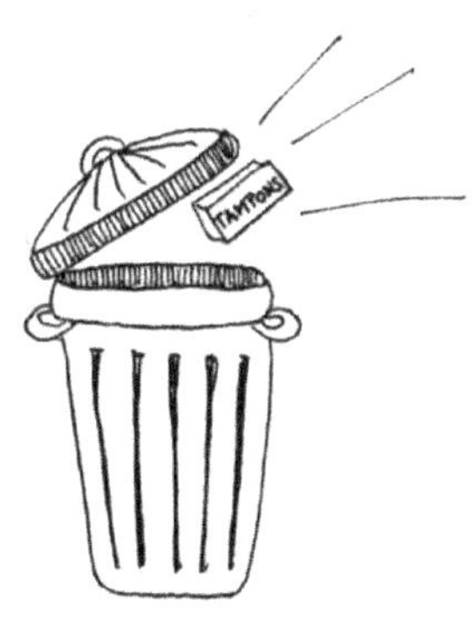

Helpful Resources and Contacts

Books

Galloping Catastrophe: Musings of a Menopausal Woman by Jennifer Kennedy. The menopause told how it really is. Laugh-out-loud funny and refreshingly honest.

Me and My Menopausal Vagina: Living with Vaginal Atrophy by Jane Lewis. An excellent guide to an all-too-common but little-talked-about symptom of the menopause. Serious, funny and informative.

Blogs

Elizabeth Carr-Ellis – journalist: www.50Sense.net

Is it just me? The day-to-day experiences of an average menopausal woman:
https://www.facebook.com/menopausalwoman

Jo – Tea & Cake for the Soul:
https://teaandcakeforthesoul.wordpress.com

Groups, Organisations and Support

Andrea Marsh – Shiatsu & Chinese Medicine Practitioner, specialising in Menopause:
www.cotswoldmenopause.co.uk

Become – Clothing designed to combat the symptoms of hot flushes and night sweats:
https://www.webecome.co.uk/

Caroline Keatinge – Nutritionist, supporting women through the Menopause and beyond:
www.carolinekeatinge.com

Clare Shepherd – Nutritional Therapist, Menopause Health Coach: www.yournewlifeplan.com

Clarity – Mindfulness, relaxation and sleep app for menopausal women: https://clarity.app/

Daisy Network – supporting women with Premature Ovarian Insufficiency: www.daisynetwork.org

Esteem - No Pause – Menopause Clothing and Solution Clothing: www.esteemmanchester.com

Health & Her – a website offering trusted expert advice and handpicked products for women experiencing perimenopause and menopause: www.healthandher.com

Henpicked – for women who weren't born yesterday:
https://henpicked.net

Joanna Meriwether, MSW – Mid-life coach and Sex Surge expert: www.JoannaMeriwether.com

Kerry Wilde – Womb Alchemist, Feminine Embodiment Coach: www.kerrywilde.com

Lauren Chiren – Menopause at Work Training Solutions and Specialist Executive Health Coaching: www.womenofacertainstage.com

Mandy Adams – Menstruality Mentor, Menopause as Rite of Passage: www.mandyadams.co.uk

MegsMenopause – an open source of information and advice on the menopause, founded by Meg Mathews: megsmenopause.com

Menomagic – Natural wellness products to maintain you through the menopause: www.menomagic.co.uk

Menopause Café – Creating spaces for conversations about menopause: www.menopausecafe.net

Menopause Matters – provides advice and support on all things menopause through their award-winning website and magazine: www.menopausematters.co.uk

Moya O'Hagan – Commercial Lead, Lancashire Women: www.lancashirewomen.org

Pausitivity: www.pausitivity.co.uk

Rachel Lankester – Midlife mentor, writer and podcast host: magnificentmidlife.com

Red School – menopause workshops (in person and online), menopause mentoring and Facebook community: www.redschool.net

Sylk Natural Lubricant – Relieves vaginal dryness and makes sex comfortable: www.sylk.co.uk

The Latte Lounge – an online platform for midlife women: www.lattelounge.co

This Girl Can – a campaign to promote sport amongst women: www.thisgirlcan.co.uk

Totes Merry Peri:
www.facebook.com/groups/353467242250396/?ref=share

Totes Inappropes:
www.facebook.com/totesinappropes123/

If you've enjoyed reading this book, you might also like the first volume in the series, *The Menopause Monologues.*

Please join us online:

Facebook: The Menopause Monologues

Twitter/Instagram: @thelittletaboo

We'd love to see you there!

Thanks

… to Michele, unfailing supporter and friend, for her loyalty, hard work and good humour.

… to Nick, for his apparently never-ending reserves of patience.

… to every single one of the fabulous women I've had the great good fortune to meet while collecting the stories for this book. You are all a lesson in strength and inspiration.

9 781916 139121